To Test or Not to Test

To Test or Not to Test

A GUIDE TO GENETIC SCREENING AND RISK

Doris Teichler Zallen

Rutgers University Press
New Brunswick, New Jersey, and London

Library of Congress Cataloging-in-Publication Data

Teichler-Zallen, Doris.
To test or not to test : a guide to genetic screening and risk / Doris Teichler Zallen.
p. cm.
Includes bibliographical references and index.
ISBN 978–0–8135–4377–2 (hardcover : alk. paper)—ISBN 978–0–8135–4378–9 (pbk. : alk. paper)
1. Genetic screening. 2. Genetic disorders—Risk factors. I. Title.
RB155.65.T45 2008
616.′042—dc22   2008000898

A British Cataloging-in-Publication record for this book is available from the British Library.

Visit our Web site: http://rutgerspress.rutgers.edu

Manufactured in the United States of America

For my mother, Bessie Teichler, our family's treasure

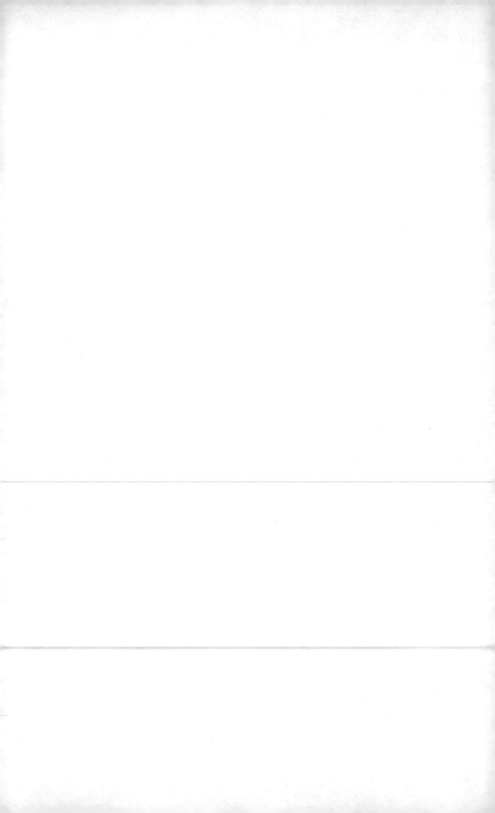

Contents

Figures and Tables

Figures

Tables

Preface

Sometimes the speed of scientific advancement is astounding. Sometimes it is frustratingly slow. And sometimes the new findings bring with them a number of perplexing personal and public issues. All of these statements fit the field of genetics. They set the stage for this book.

At the turn of the twentieth century, the rediscovery of Mendel's laws provided the spark for the investigation of inheritance in a variety of animals and plants. Human beings, for the most part, were left out (as subjects) of this upsurge in genetic research. Humans are difficult to study using Mendelian approaches. They have too few children, their generation time is too long, and they stubbornly refuse to reproduce with designated partners for the purpose of answering research questions. But by the turn of the twenty-first century, the situation had changed. Scientists had discovered how to isolate and study the genetic material directly. This catapulted humans to prominence as research subjects. Just by studying human genetic material, human DNA, it became possible to search out genes and to design ways to understand how these genes function and, occasionally, malfunction. We are now experiencing a tide of discovery that, on a daily basis, floods our scientific journals—as well as the popular media—with new genetic insights. Genetic tests of all sorts have been developed. These can probe the human genetic material and determine the status of whole chromosomes, parts of chromosomes, and of individual genes themselves. The number of such tests that are already available is considerable. This number will continue to grow as the boom in genetic research continues.

A beneficial application of all this genetic knowledge, as it makes its way into doctors' offices and clinics, is the improvement of human health and well-being. This is accomplished by using the research findings to prevent disorders from occurring, or to provide effective treatments and even cures if they do occur. Here the pace of progress, while impressive, is not as spectacular as the pace of scientific discovery. Effective medical interventions have been slow to develop. Complicating the mismatch between knowledge and intervention are a number of historical, ethical, social, and policy issues that have long bedeviled the world of genetics. The end result is that decisions about the use of genetic tests can be difficult, even daunting.

For some years now, a main goal of my own program of research has been to disentangle—and to identify—the many elements associated with the genetic-test decision process. My previous book, *Does It Run in the Family: A Consumer's Guide to DNA Testing for Genetic Disorders*, emphasized genetic testing for the rare disorders. Rare disorders are those conditions brought on when a single gene fails to function properly. The field of genetics research has expanded its range, so that the newest genetic tests are able to identify genes that are in some way associated with common disorders. Having a flaw in one of these genes makes it more likely that a person will develop a particular disorder. It is these newest tests, the ones now on the genetic frontier but destined soon to become workhorses within the health-care community, that form the main focus of my current research and of this book.

To Test or Not to Test is intended to be useful to several different audiences. For those individuals who are faced with the prospect of a genetic test, it provides a template that can guide the decision process. For health-care professionals (many of whom do not yet have experience with the newest genetic tests), it should help to reveal the personal values, family dilemmas, and societal realities associated with such testing. And for those serving in governmental agencies, professional organizations, and private companies, it will point out areas in which there is a need to shape protective policies.

Acknowledgments

Investigating the many different dimensions of genetic testing is a challenging task. The research on which this book is based was begun during a sabbatical leave that I was able to spend at the Center for Ethics and Humanities in the Life Sciences at Michigan State University. The Center provided a rich interdisciplinary setting in which the humanistic issues surrounding the new modes of genetic testing for common disorders could be teased out and evaluated. I also had access to Michigan State's active genetic counseling program, where many of the newest genetic tests are already in routine use. The work done there was further extended by a grant from the National Endowment for the Humanities (FT-51474–03). This grant made possible an analogous exploration of those same genetic-testing issues in the United Kingdom. In the United States, financial factors and fears about the loss of health insurance can sometimes mask other types of personal issues. Because of its national health system, such factors are largely absent in the U.K., allowing for somewhat more emphasis on personal and family issues. A Dean's Faculty Fellowship from the College of Liberal Arts and Human Sciences at Virginia Tech made it possible for me to write up the research findings. I am indebted to these institutions for providing resources that were crucial in first launching this work and then in helping to bring it to fruition.

In the intervening period, as the data-gathering phase of the study moved into high gear, many voluntary health organizations, patient-interest groups, and informal Web-based groups called this study to the attention of their members. Thanks to their help, I was able to reach individuals from many different parts of the country and in many different life situations, including those who, for a variety of reasons, were not within the orbit of the health-care system. I was privileged to be able to speak with—and learn from— about one hundred individuals who generously shared their personal experiences with me. I am grateful for their willingness to contribute their own valuable time to this study, and wish to especially thank them for their candor and their unflinching consideration of the sensitive genetic-testing issues they faced.

I had the opportunity to become aware of a wide spectrum of consumer issues through in-depth conversations with Charlotte Augst (CancerBACUP, U.K.), Michelle Barclay (Cancer Breakthrough, U.K.), Diane Barnett (Contact a Family, U.K.), Jane Fior (Cancer Counseling Trust, U.K.), Sue Friedman (FORCE: Facing Our Risk of Cancer Empowered, U.S.), Pritti Mehta and Parul Vansadia (Genetic Interest Group, U.K.), and Michael Retsky (Colon Cancer Alliance, U.S.).

The interviews with consumers and consumer advocates were augmented by interviews with individuals who are on the front lines of genetic testing in several professional capacities. Genetic counselors, working within many types of medical settings, form a vital bridge between the realm of science and the individuals in need of information and help. I was fortunate indeed to be able to benefit from the vast experience of Melissa Barber, Rashmi Chikarmane, Libby Couchon, Leigh Ann Flore, Cara Flynn, Ruth Glew, Jill Goldman, Ann Jewell, Steven Keiles, Susan LaRusse Eckert, Erin Linnenbringer, Elissa Levin, Annette Patterson, Nancie Petrucelli, Gladys Rosenthal, Hetal Sheth, Charlene Shultz, Cecile Skrzynia, Lisa Susswein, Susan Tinley, Elizabeth Varga, and Rebecca Zoller.

Scientists working at the lab bench, physicians caring for patients, and scholars exploring both the human dimensions and the public-policy dimensions of genetic testing helped me to understand these real-world aspects of genetic testing. I was able to draw on the expertise of Samuel Barondes, David Brook, Angus Clarke, Bard Cosman, Jon Emery, Peter Harper, Shirley Hodgson, Ruth Itzhaki, Louise Izatt, Simon Lovestone, James Mackay, Usha Menon, Stephan Moll, Michael Netzloff, Elizabeth Petty, Kimberly Quaid, Susan Winter, Ashok Amin, Lee Blecher, Catherine Haga, Joni Kaiser, William Silverstone, Joan Austoker, Jill Elfenbein, Lynne Hodgson, Ryan Phelan, and Martin Richards.

Tammy Stevers, Mary Cato, and Chris Hays provided outstanding assistance in data collection, organization, and the identification of additional resources for consumers. Bard Cosman took special pains to review the manuscript for medical accuracy. My most caring critics—Richard Zallen, Jennifer Zallen, and Avi Zallen—were pressed into service to review the text for clarity. I took much of the advice I was given, but not all. So for remaining errors in substance, style, and syntax, I have only myself to blame.

And, finally, I am incredibly grateful for the love and encouragement of my family throughout this project and for the special gifts of Robyn's kisses, Ben's hugs, and Megan's sweet smiles.

Important Note

Throughout this book, I will be drawing from the actual experiences of real individuals who have faced the issues and challenges involved in genetic testing. In order to protect the privacy of these generous individuals who were willing to allow us to look into their lives, I am not using their real names and I have changed details of their family histories and their stories. So if you think that you recognize someone, you will be mistaken.

The main goal of this book is to suggest a template or guide for decision making about genetic testing. There is no intention to endorse any of the specific decisions made by the individuals who have contributed to this study, whether those decisions were to have or not to have genetic testing, to share or not to share genetic information, or to choose or to reject a particular form of treatment or a particular means of prevention. Each of us must make our own decision, in the context of our own life, with input from qualified medical professionals.

To Test or Not to Test

CHAPTER ONE

Introduction: Genetic Tests Are Different

An Old Joke

It seems that two boys, very good friends, each had gotten a pony for his birthday. They were delighted, of course. The only problem was that they found it impossible to tell the two animals apart. Once, one boy put a bell around the neck of his pony only to discover that his friend had done the same thing. The other boy had the idea of putting a red ribbon on his pony's tail but then found that his friend had also done exactly that. Finally, in desperation, they decided to measure the two animals very carefully, hand over hand. Sure enough, the white pony was two hands taller than the brown one.

We don't give it a second thought. It all seems so ordinary. Whether we are perched on the end of an examining table in a doctor's office or shivering in a skimpy gown in a hospital room, we know that we are going to be tested in some way or other. Tests are a standard part of modern medicine. They are what we have come to expect and even demand. And so, depending on our health needs, we willingly undergo tests of our blood and urine, our vision and hearing. We have stress tests and strep tests, biopsies and bronchoscopies, mammographies, endoscopies, colonoscopies. We seek out tests with names so complicated that we can only refer to them by their initials: PET, ECG, CT, MRI. From head to toe, inside and out, in every way possible, we are tested.

The newest additions to the medical-test toolbox are genetic tests. Genetic tests are designed to explore those tiny hereditary units—our genes—hidden away in each of the cells in our bodies. These tests probe the threadlike substance, DNA, of which genes are made, looking for any flaws. As we have come to know, even a small change in the genetic material can cause health problems. In some cases, these problems can show up right away; in other cases, they may make themselves known much later on in life.

At first glance, there doesn't seem to be much difference between genetic tests and other types of medical tests. After all, undergoing any medical test can sometimes be quite troubling and can create anxiety, and the results can produce extreme distress for those who receive bad news. In fact, like the two ponies in that old joke recalled above, genetic tests—those tests designed to reveal flaws in our genes—are different from other kinds of medical tests. And genetic information is different from other kinds of medical information. What makes genetic tests and the information they provide about our genes so special?

First of all, there is the scope of genetic information. Genes are inherited. They are passed along from parents to children to grandchildren. Genes are shared in families. A genetic test that provides information about one person can, at the same time, indicate to others in the family that they too may have the same gene. More than any other type of testing, a genetic test of a single individual is actually a test of a whole family. Receiving a test result may create an obligation to transmit one's personal information to relatives outside of the immediate family—something that we seldom feel pressured to do with other medical tests. Studies have shown that information gathered from genetic tests has created rifts in families as people struggle to understand and share this information. Sometimes relatives blame one another for being the source of a flawed gene, or try to find out just who the gene for a disorder "came from." Such intense, sometimes even violent, reactions rarely arise with other types of medical tests.

Genetic tests can offer glimpses into—or predictions about—the future. Unlike other types of tests that are snapshots of a person's health at the moment of testing, a genetic test can alert people who are perfectly healthy right now that they may be at significant risk for having a particular disorder develop in the years or decades ahead. A genetic test is like looking into a crystal ball to see what health problems one may be destined to face. Such a prediction can prove to be extremely unsettling.

These two features are further complicated by the special position that genes occupy in contemporary life. Other types of medical tests are seen as indicators of health or illness, but usually they don't carry with them any value judgment about the worth or merit of the person being tested. Not so for genetic tests. Genes have come to be regarded as very important defining elements of who we are and what we will become. A pendulum has swung back and forth over recent history between nature and nurture—between regarding biological influences or environmental influences as most important. That pendulum now has swung far to the nature—the genetic—side of things. The reasons for this are complex, but a main factor seems to be the steady diet of overly enthusiastic genetic news that comes to us nowadays through the media. In the hoopla surrounding research efforts such as the Human Genome Project (the international endeavor, concluded in 2003, to find the complete chemical sequence of all the human genes), scientists have referred to the human genetic makeup as the "holy grail" or the "book of life." This hyperbole has found a home in the popular press. We constantly read or hear stories that feature dramatic new findings about genes and their connections to a variety of diseases and human characteristics—supposedly even for traits such as using good grammar and taking risks. These stories perpetuate the message that it is our genes, and our genes alone, that determine who we are. With this steady drumbeat of scientific and journalistic excess, the message is repeated over and over again. It's no wonder that we have come to regard ourselves as exclusively defined by our genes. It's also no wonder that environmental contributions that regulate, alter, and neutralize gene function—hormone levels, lifestyle choices, exposure to such things as workplace chemicals, toxins, and infectious diseases—have slipped into the shadows. In this climate, a genetic test result indicating the presence of a flawed gene can make people themselves feel flawed. They can feel diminished, tainted.

Genetic information is also different because of the way that it has been misused in the past. The history here is that of the eugenics movement—or eugenics movements, really, since they arose in different countries and led to different kinds of governmental policies. These movements got their start from the ideas of Francis Galton in England at the end of the nineteenth century. Galton noted that "characteristics cling to families" and he advocated the development of public policies that promoted the reproduction of those who were biologically "superior" (this is also known as positive eugenics) and limited the reproduction of those who were viewed as biologically "inferior" (or negative eugenics). Keep in mind that, to Galton and other supporters of his ideas, biologically superior meant getting your college degree at Oxford or Cambridge; biologically inferior meant being poor or uneducated or unskilled. The eugenics movements really took off around the world at the turn of the twentieth century with the popularization of Mendel's laws of inheritance. Now, personal characteristics could be tied to discrete units—what we today call "genes." It was no longer just some amorphous "biology," but specific units of heredity that could now be held responsible for bringing about desirable or undesirable traits. Rather quickly, absurd ideas spread that almost any behavioral attribute (such as intelligence or tidiness) or social problem (for example, poverty and criminality) could be tied to specific individual genes. Unfortunately, many of these misguided ideas were used to drive the creation of governmental eugenic policies.

When it comes to eugenic policies, Nazi Germany was certainly the moral abyss. But, in less extreme forms, these policies flourished elsewhere. They were even enthusiastically pursued in the United States, where laws regarding eugenics were enacted in dozens of states. The positive-eugenics approach took the relatively benign form of holding large-family and small-family competitions at state fairs, where blue ribbons were awarded to "fitter families." The negative-eugenics approach was another matter. It was two-pronged. One prong was directed at foreigners. It was aimed at keeping out the bad genes by restricting the entry into this country of immigrant groups that were regarded as genetically inferior. The other prong was directed at citizens within the United States who were considered genetically inferior. For them, there was involuntary sterilization. What drove eugenic sterilizations into high gear was the 1927 U.S. Supreme Court decision of *Buck v. Bell*, which declared such sterilizations acceptable under the Constitution. Records indicate that at least 60,000 such involuntary sterilizations—but likely many more—were carried out in the years that followed. These eugenic policies fell into well-earned disrepute after the Second World War because of their lack of scientific validity and the clear evidence of their painful human cost. The laws themselves were abandoned in most places by the mid-1970s. Whether or not people can recite the details of eugenics history, the fact that there have been instances of being punished for your genes—of suffering harm or discrimination or death because of your genes—still lurks in the background whenever genetic matters are raised. In practical terms, this translates into the fear that if a genetic test points out some inherited deficiency, a person could be denied insurance or jobs, educational opportunities or government services. Even worse, such penalties might also be directed at others in the family who, though not tested themselves, could be marked as sharing the same genes by virtue of their family relationship.

All these points of difference, along with the harsh realities that can accompany them, place genetic testing into a category separate from other types of medical tests. The time may come when genetic information will no longer have the special place that it has right now. But for the present and for the foreseeable future, we need to think through the ifs, hows, whens, and whys of genetic testing both for ourselves and for our families.

The Next Generation of Genetic Tests

The range of genetic tests that are available has been expanding over the last decades. In the 1960s, the first tests to come along were able to examine the human chromosomes. (Chromosomes are the relatively large multigene structures that are visible under a microscope. Individual genes are much smaller and cannot be seen with a microscope.) These tests were effective in identifying individuals who had disorders resulting from an incorrect number of chromosomes. Usually, there are 23 pairs of chromosomes in a cell. For individuals with Down syndrome, there is an extra chromosome 21. For individuals with Klinefelter syndrome, there is an extra X chromosome. The early tests could identify individuals with these and other types of chromosomal disorders. But since each chromosome contains many different genes, these first tests could not shed light on the status of any individual gene.

Tests for specific genes were first introduced in the 1970s. These were indirect; they looked for the presence or absence of products for which a specific gene is responsible. Tests that probed the DNA directly came next. At first, these DNA genetic tests were used in situations in which the presence of a single flawed gene (or gene pair) could, by itself, bring on a serious health problem. There are many disorders of this kind, although each individual disorder tends to be rare. They include Huntington disease, sickle-cell anemia, neurofibromatosis, and cystic fibrosis. Much of the current interest in the personal, family, and social issues surrounding DNA testing began with our experience with genetic tests for these disorders.

Recent advances in genetics, spurred on by the wealth of information gathered through the Human Genome Project, have led to a whole new generation of genetic tests. These new tests look for genetic flaws associated with common disorders such as cancer or Alzheimer's disease. It turns out that most of the common disorders—the major health problems that afflict us—are brought on by a combination of many different genes interacting in complicated ways with a variety of environmental factors. Scientists and physicians are only beginning to understand the rogues' gallery of genes and the environmental factors responsible for each disorder. What is known is that a flaw in any one of the constellation of genes can increase the chance that a particular disorder could occur later on in a person's life. However, since other genes and environmental factors are also involved, there is no certainty, even with a flawed gene present, that the disorder will ever develop. (A brief background on these tests can be found in chapter 2.)

Given the interest of the medical community in diagnosing and treating the common health problems that take such a terrible toll in human suffering and loss of life, these new genetic tests are receiving a great deal of interest and attention. Predictions are that this form of genetic testing—testing for your heightened susceptibility to develop certain diseases—will be incorporated rapidly into standard medical care and that it will change the face of modern medicine. The view is that medical care in the twenty-first century will rely heavily on genetic information to discover the specific disorders each of us is likely to fall prey to, the ones to which we are especially susceptible. Unlike the Greek tragedies in which it is impossible to escape one's fate, once we learn of our susceptibilities, we might be able to take steps to prevent those disorders from ever developing, much as we build levees in low-lying areas to keep out the sea water. Of course, even the best attempts at prevention can be swept away by an array of environmental and other factors. Still, at the very least, the tests could help us and our physicians be on the alert to diagnose specific disorders in their earliest stages when they can be dealt with more effectively. Because many people (and/or their physicians) will wish to know the illnesses to which they are most susceptible, there is expected to be much interest in the research community in developing these genetic tests, in testing laboratories in marketing these tests, and by pharmaceutical companies, in the discovery of treatments and genetic cures.

Whether or not this new genetic age ends up being as revolutionary as anticipated, in the years ahead most of us will be presented with the opportunity to have genetic tests that can indicate our susceptibility to a wide range of health problems. Some laboratories and corporations are aggressively marketing their genetic tests to physicians and, even more aggressively, to the public through ads in magazines and on television and on the Internet.

Some companies are marketing "genetic tests" that promote their own corporate skin products and dietary supplements. People are feeling pressured to jump on the genetic-test bandwagon.

As we have seen, genetic tests are different from standard medical tests and have far-ranging implications for individuals and for their families. These tests should not be regarded as automatic or routine. Each of us must decide for ourselves whether or not we wish to undergo this form of testing. As discussed in this book, there are circumstances in which an individual might well decide to be tested. But there are also circumstances in which an individual might well decide not to be tested. The problem is how to decide.

Making Decisions about Genetic Tests for Susceptibility to Disorders

How, indeed, do we decide about having a genetic test? This book is the result of a research effort designed to help answer this question. In general, it is usually appropriate to turn to experts, to draw on their experience and gain their advice. That is what we have done here. Over 150 interviews were conducted with experts on the front lines of genetic testing. One-third of these interviews were with genetic professionals: researchers, physicians, and genetic counselors. These individuals are associated with leading genetics centers in the United States as well as in Canada and the United Kingdom. Individually and collectively, they have a wealth of knowledge about genetic testing. They were able to describe how the new DNA tests for common disorders are being used in genetics clinics and in doctors' offices. They provided a broad overview of the degree to which these newest tests have been taken up by the medical community and how willing patients are to make use of them. These interviews were supplemented by reports of the new DNA tests written by genetics researchers and published in leading scientific journals.

There is another set of experts whose voices are often unheard, but whose knowledge and insight are substantial. These are the people who have already faced the decision about whether or not to use these tests because of concerns about health problems in their own lives. About 100 such individuals—for want of a better term, I will call them consumers—were interviewed. I reached them through genetics clinics and patient-support groups. They were concerned about health problems such as cancer, Alzheimer's disease, and iron overload disorders that had entered their lives or the lives of their family members. These people, who graciously consented to share their stories, come from a wide spectrum of social and economic circumstances. They have different religious preferences and ethnic backgrounds. During the interviews they were not asked to respond to a fixed set of survey questions. Instead, they were invited to share their experiences. As a result, different topics arose and were pursued further in the course of each interview. These consumers described not only how they became aware of the genetic tests but how they made their decisions. In several cases, it was possible to explore the different decisions made by members of the same family. Most of the participants in this study were in a position to judge, with the benefit of hindsight, how satisfied they were with the choices they had made or what regrets or misgivings they had about their decisions. These interviews yielded oral histories that are a rich source of information about the ways people think about genetic testing and how they make their individual and very personal decisions.

Four different areas of genetic testing form the focal points for this research. These areas were chosen so that we would have sufficient depth of experience from both professionals and consumers to permit general conclusions to emerge. The selection of these areas was made on the basis of the genetic tests for susceptibility that are currently available and on the spectrum of issues that surround such testing. We needed to explore testing that involves men as well as women, older as well as younger people, testing where treatments are available for the disorder and where they are not, and where there are different means of prevention. Thus, the types of genetic testing that we will be using as our examples are breast/ovarian cancer (these two seemingly different disorders are, in fact, closely connected), colon cancer (the form known as HNPCC, hereditary non-polyposis colon cancer, or Lynch syndrome), late-onset Alzheimer's disease, and hereditary hemochromatosis. Hemochromatosis is less well known because it is hard to recognize and is underdiagnosed by the medical community. Nonetheless, the gene flaws associated with it are quite common, especially in the Caucasian population, and its impact on human lives is substantial. And although in the recent past Alzheimer's disease genetic testing has typically been restricted to research studies, such testing is now available to the wider public.

The examples used here are intended not only to be useful to those concerned about these four illnesses, but are also intended to serve as models to illustrate how to make decisions in the future about any genetic test for susceptibility. Researchers are identifying genetic connections to a vast variety of other diseases such as diabetes, prostate cancer, high blood pressure, heart disease, rheumatoid arthritis, macular degeneration, inflammatory bowel disease, and bipolar disorder. Once these connections are confirmed, genetic tests for susceptibility will follow. The examples mentioned here represent just a small sample of the wide range of genetic tests that will eventually become available.

Based on these different strands of expertise, and building on the foundation of related previous work dealing with genetic testing for rare disorders, we find that four elements figure into decisions about DNA testing for common diseases. These elements can be expressed as four key questions that need to be considered as any decision about genetic testing is thought through:

1. Am I at a higher risk for this disease than other people?
2. Will the test give me useful information?
3. Is this the right time in my life to be taking this test?
4. Will the advantages gained from having the genetic information outweigh the disadvantages?

A "yes" answer to all of these questions should be a prerequisite for deciding to get tested. A "no" answer to any of these questions should lead one to forgo testing or, at least, to put it on the back burner until the situation changes sufficiently to convert a "no" into a "yes." But determining the answers to each of these questions is no easy task. Chapters 3 through 6 will explore each of these questions in turn, in greater detail. Chapter 7 will point out resources that you may want to use as you think matters through and make your decision. Chapter 8 shows how this same decision-making template applies to other types of genetic testing as well.

The oral history interviews also provided a means of recognizing the educational, legal, and other barriers that stand in the way of genetic medicine. These barriers, and general policy recommendations to overcome them, will be discussed in chapter 9.

Before we begin, it would be helpful to have some basic background about genes, how they may be connected to potential for disease, and how the new DNA tests work. That will be our mission in the next chapter.

CHAPTER TWO

A Brief Overview of Susceptibility-Gene Testing

Some basic knowledge of the scientific aspects is helpful as you proceed on the path to a decision about genetic testing. But to acquire this knowledge, you don't have to enter a graduate program in genetics. This chapter provides a general overview of susceptibility-gene testing that should be sufficient to assist with your decision making. (For those readers who wish to go more deeply into the science, a tutorial on genetics can be found in the Appendix. In addition, the Resources section points to other materials that provide further scientific background.)

What Are "Susceptibility Genes"?

Despite the fact that we use the word "gene" all the time, scientists have still been unable to come up with a simple definition—because genes can take on many roles. They act in many different ways in the life of the individual to ensure that the body develops properly over the lifespan and to ensure that numerous chemical activities, necessary to maintain life, are carried out efficiently. So coming up with a simple or comprehensive definition for the gene is difficult.

Though estimates differ, let us assume that we humans have about 25,000 different genes. Some of the genes in this collection can have a large impact on how we function. They act to enable key substances to be made or vital functions to be carried out. Other genes have a much less decisive role on their own. Instead, they act as a team, in combination with other genes, each one making a modest contribution to the formation of a body structure or the carrying out of a job or an activity. Environmental factors such as diet, lifestyle, exposure to infections or toxins—and many others that we don't yet know or understand—interact with genes. In various ways, environmental factors can have an effect on increasing or inhibiting gene activity. It might be best just to think of genes in general as units that have the ability to make a contribution—large or small, on their own or in response to outside signals—that help bring about the overall harmonious functioning of every living being.

The same gene can vary in small ways from person to person. Most of these variations are unimportant. They have no effect at all on how the gene functions. However, other variations are more serious. These do affect how well the gene functions. This type of small flaw or defect—what scientists would call a *mutation*—throws a monkey wrench into what otherwise would be harmonious functioning and can create a dissonance that can reveal itself in different ways.

If the flaw or mutation (and I use these terms interchangeably) occurs in one of those genes that has a large impact on its own, an important bodily task may not be carried out at all. This failure to function properly may introduce all manner of mayhem and cause serious health problems that frequently come on during the first years of life. Examples here would be Tay-Sachs disease, cystic fibrosis, spinal-muscular atrophy, and sickle-cell anemia. We generally call these "single-gene disorders" because the health consequences can be attributed to a flaw in a particular gene.

But for disorders connected with susceptibility genes, the flaw is present in one of those genes that typically works as part of a team, in partnership with several other genes. When one of these team-player genes is flawed, the task for which they are all responsible may still be carried out, but in a slightly substandard manner. Perhaps because one such gene has a mutation that turns it into a bit of a slacker, waste products of chemical reactions in the body will not be removed with full efficiency. Very slowly and over long periods of time, these wastes could accumulate to levels high enough to interfere with the way the body functions. Or perhaps, in the presence of a flawed gene, there will be a decreased ability to repair the damage that continually occurs to the genetic material itself as we grow and age. Over time, this could make it more likely for an unlucky normal cell to accumulate so much damage that it is transformed into a cancer cell (and the start of a tumor).

Even with such a flawed gene present, it can be decades before any health problem shows up. And, depending on circumstances, no problem may occur at all. These circumstances include the way a particular mutation affects how the gene functions (different mutations can have different effects, some very mild and almost unnoticeable), how much the gene actually contributed when it was functioning properly, the level of function by the other genes that are working together with it, and by all those outside influences that we lump together as environmental factors. It is possible that those other genes might be able to work a little harder and compensate for the reduced effort by the slacker gene. It is also possible, even in the presence of a flawed gene, that with the right assortment of environmental factors, no health problem may ever occur. Of course, it is also possible that, given a different set of environmental factors, health problems can result even without any known genetic involvement. Overall then, the presence of this type of mutant gene may raise the risk of developing a particular health problem—may make someone more prone to develop that problem—but does not guarantee it will occur. And, because of the involvement of environmental factors, the health problem can occur even in the absence of any known mutation.

To sum up, we give the name "susceptibility gene" to a gene that, when it is flawed, increases the chance that a specific health problem will develop later on in life. It turns out that susceptibility genes are associated with the major diseases afflicting our society. In this book we are concerned with genetic tests for these common, and often very serious, illnesses.

The New Genetic Tests

Genetic testing is done to figure out if a particular gene is functioning properly or if that gene possesses a mutation that alters its ability to function. Genetic testing of this type has been underway for several decades. The first tests centered on genes that, when mutated, bring on the single-gene disorders. The newest genetic tests, the ones that are in the vanguard of the anticipated genetic revolution in medicine, are those for susceptibility genes. You can imagine that it is not an easy task to identify those genes that are susceptibility genes because each one interacts with other genes and with a variety of environmental factors. Unraveling it all will certainly take some time. Genetic researchers have developed a number of tricks of the trade that are allowing them to find out which genes in our genetic inventory are the ones associated with a predisposition to a specific health problem, and whether any flaws are present in those genes. The first susceptibility genes that have been found are the ones that, for various reasons, have been easier to spot against the din of genetic activity.

From the susceptibility gene tests now available I have selected four disorders to serve as our standard "database." We will use these four disorders as models from which to draw general insights about genetic testing. These insights should apply to any type of susceptibility-gene testing, including tests that are now in use, those in the pipeline, and those to come in the future. The four representative disorders are listed in table 2.1. For two of them (hemochromatosis and Alzheimer's disease) there is only one susceptibility gene currently known. For the other two (breast/ovarian cancer and nonpolyposis colon cancer), several susceptibility genes have already been identified. Sometimes only one or a few mutations have been found within those genes. Sometimes many different mutations have been found. Table 2.1 also includes the environmental factors known to contribute to these diseases.

All that is needed for a genetic test is a sample of one's genetic material. Because genetic material occurs in every part of the body, the sample can be collected by drawing a small amount of blood into a tube or by removing tiny bits of tissue by gently swabbing the inside of the mouth. The substance of which the

Table 2.1. Representative Common Disorders with Their Genetic and Environmental Influences

Disorder	Features	Known Susceptibility Genes	Mutations or Variations	Known Environmental Factors
Hemochromatosis (type 1)	Very high iron absorption and storage in body organs, which can lead to diabetes mellitus, cirrhosis, liver cancer, and other problems	HFE gene (Both gene copies must have a mutation for the symptoms to appear.)	C282Y, H63D	Diets high in iron or iron supplements; alcohol consumption
Breast/ovarian cancer	Cancer in the breast and/or the ovaries. Other types of cancer, including prostate cancer, can also result.	BRCA1 BRCA2 (These genes help repair damage in DNA.)	Many mutations have been found. Some are specific to families or occur more frequently in certain heritage groups.	Menstruation before age 12, first pregnancy after 30, or menopause after 55; hormone replacement therapy
Hereditary non-polyposis colon cancer (HNPCC), also called Lynch syndrome	Colon cancer. Cancer of the ovary, the endometrium, and the digestive track can also occur	MLH1 MSH2 MSH6 PMS2 (These genes help repair DNA mismatch errors.)	Many different mutations have been found in these genes	Diet, tobacco use
Alzheimer's disease, late-onset form	Progressive dementia associated with structural changes (plaques and neurofibrillary tangles) in the brain	Apo-E (This gene helps with the removal of lipids.)	ε-4 form of the Apo-E gene	Head injury, some childhood infections

genes are constructed—DNA—can then be isolated and examined in the laboratory.

It is crucial to keep in mind that even if a flaw is found, it does not mean that the person is certain to come down with the illness at some point in the future. It only means that the individual has a heightened susceptibility to that illness, that he or she has a greater chance than average of developing the illness or condition with which the flawed gene is associated. On the other hand, a test result that shows the absence of any flaws in a gene is not a guarantee that the person will be spared that particular health problem. It just means that one's risk for the illness—whichever illness it is—is no more and no less than what you would expect for the whole population.

Patterns of Inheritance

People who are found to have mutant susceptibility genes often wonder how they have come to have them. Well, somewhere in the distant past, a mutation occurred in a gene in a reproductive cell—egg or sperm—much as a typo can occur in a document. Since genes are inherited, they are passed on from one generation to the next. If a mutant gene is present, it can be passed on along with the other genes. We all contain two copies of each of our genes. Each parent contributes half of his or her own personal gene inventory to each child; one copy of each gene passes through the sperm and one copy of each gene passes through the egg. So, at each pregnancy, there is a 50 percent chance that the mutant gene will be passed along from the parent who has that gene to the child.

For two of the examples featured in this book—breast/ovarian cancer and nonpolyposis colon cancer—having one copy of a mutant susceptibility gene is sufficient to make an individual more susceptible to the disorder. For another of our examples—hemochromatosis—both genes of the pair have to contain a mutation in order for an individual to become more susceptible.

For our fourth example, Alzheimer's disease, the degree of susceptibility rises if one member of the gene pair contains the mutant
gene and is higher still if both do.

It is always important to keep in mind that

- other genes and environmental factors may be such that the
  disorder may not develop even when the flawed gene (or
  genes) is present, and
- people without the flawed gene can still develop the disorder.
  These illnesses can—and, in fact, most often do—arise in
  individuals who have no genetic predisposition.

Now, let's get to work. With this background, let's turn our attention
to each of the questions that must be addressed before we can make
an informed decision about whether a particular susceptibility-
gene test is right for us.

CHAPTER THREE

Am I at a Higher Risk for This Disease than Other People?

Discovering an Inherited Health Problem

I am like the Rosetta stone for my family.

I had been having symptoms for years and the main thing that bothered me was irregular heartbeats. They sort of came on and then would go away. So, I consulted a cardiologist and went through a whole series of tests and he found nothing. Anyway, long story short, it got to where my heart was beating so irregularly that it almost incapacitated me in terms of moving around. I went to see a new doctor, a family doctor, whose office was nearby. She gave me a physical and about a week later I got a letter from her saying that I might have hemochromatosis. I went back to her office for more tests and, sure enough, that's what I had. It's hard to pronounce and I'd never heard of it before. What was happening was that my blood was overloaded with iron and some of that iron was being deposited in the organs of my body, including my heart. Somehow, this strange-sounding disease was the explanation for all the heart problems I was experiencing and some of my other health problems as well. I wasn't a giant overload case, but it was very significant.

I thought, am I getting the iron from my well water? So I bought a very expensive water test. It was about $175 to test for all sorts of components in the water. It came back that I have about as pure a water as you can find anywhere, so I wasn't getting the iron from there. It was coming from the food I was eating!

What I learned from looking around on the Internet was that this disease is hereditary. The rest of my family—my two younger brothers, my daughter, even my cousin—may be at risk too.

—Todd B., age sixty

The physician's toolbox is filled with all sorts of tests for a huge array of health problems. It is not realistic, affordable, or even wise to undergo testing for every kind of health problem that might possibly come our way in the course of a lifetime. And, as a practical matter, there aren't enough resources in the medical community to test all of us for every possible illness that we might eventually develop.

Genetic tests for mutations that increase our susceptibility to a disease—the very tests that we are concerned with here—are among the latest additions to this assortment of medical tests. To find out if you are an appropriate candidate for any one of these genetic tests, the first thing you need to determine is whether there is any medical reason for you to have such a test. The major medical reason would be that you are at a higher risk for a particular disorder than other people. If it's possible that you are at higher risk, then you should go on to consider the three other questions that are part of the genetic-test decision process. If you are not— that is, if your risk for that specific disorder appears to be the same as it is for anyone else in the general population—then there may be no need to pursue the option of genetic testing for susceptibility to that disorder.

The "average risk" for a specific disease expresses the overall chance that an individual will develop a particular disorder during the course of his or her lifetime. This is an estimate, one that is based on the number of cases that have been observed in the population in the past. This average risk number can vary somewhat, of course, in different genders, geographic areas, or, sometimes, ethnic groups. The risks that the average person faces for the health problems that are serving as our examples here are listed in table 3.1. Also in that table are the estimated risks associated with the presence of susceptibility-gene mutations. As we can see, the presence of a mutant susceptibility gene (or mutant genes for hemochromatosis) substantially raises one's risk above that for the general population. In the case of Alzheimer's disease, this increase can be relatively

Table 3.1. Increased Risk Associated with Genetic Susceptibility

Disorder	Lifetime Risk for Someone in the General Population	Lifetime Risk for Someone with Known Mutations
Hemochromatosis (type 1)	About 0.4%	About 2% for those with two copies of C282Y, about 1% for those with one C282Y gene and one H63D gene
Breast cancer	About 12% of women	Between 40% and 80%, depending on the mutation
Ovarian cancer	About 1%	Between 20% and 40%, depending on the mutation
Colon cancer	About 6%	Between 60% and 80%, depending on the mutation
Alzheimer's disease, late-onset form	About 5% by age 70, about 30% by age 85	About 10–25% by age 70, depending on number of ε-4 genes; about 50–75% by age 85, depending on number of ε-4 genes

modest depending on the age of the individual and the number of ε-4 genes present.

Is My Risk Average or Above Average?

So how can we figure out if our risk may be higher than the average (or population) risk? How can we determine whether there might be a flawed susceptibility gene lurking somewhere in our own family that, if we inherited it, would put us at a higher risk? This is not an easy task since these new genetic tests provide information regarding susceptibility to health problems that are very common. Because these health problems are so common, they can appear in any family—just by chance—and sometimes more frequently in some families—again, just by chance—without any hereditary factors being involved at all. As we saw in chapter 2, environmental factors play an important role in triggering the onset of these common illnesses.

In seeking to determine if there might be a hereditary component present in your family that increases your susceptibility to a disorder, the first port of call is the family doctor. After all, the family medical history gathered in your medical file is the best resource for identifying patterns of illness. Indeed, several of the people interviewed in this study were alerted to the possibility of a hereditary predisposition by their own doctors. In one case it was a doctor, taking a family history, who noted the relatively frequent occurrence of colon cancer in a family.

> I went to a dermatologist that I hadn't been to before. He took my family history before he started his examination. He asked how did your mother die, how did your grandmother die, the whole thing. And he wheeled around on his stool and said something about the number of deaths from colon cancer. . . . I knew my grandmother on my mother's side had died when my mother was ten, and I knew she had cancer. And my mother had had colon cancer. And then my sister had colon cancer when she was about thirty-two. They thought she had a tumor or cyst on her ovary, and when they operated they found it was not that, it was cancer. I hadn't given it a whole lot of thought even though it had been in the family. I was busy raising kids and working, and so I hadn't given it a lot of thought.

In another case, it was a genetic counselor, speaking with a woman who had come in for prenatal genetic testing of her fetus during a pregnancy, who noted a number of breast cancer cases in the family pedigree that she was putting together during the counseling session.

Unfortunately, we cannot rely exclusively on the medical profession to identify individuals who may be at higher risk for particular illnesses. All too often in the restricted time of an office visit, especially if there is an urgent problem at hand to deal with, a complete family history is not taken, or it is taken but is not examined closely enough to identify any patterns of illness. Frequently, the family history that has been gathered is perfunctory. Sometimes the right questions are not asked so that, for example, no information is requested about the father's side of the family when evaluating the occurrence of breast or ovarian cancer even though susceptibility genes, including those for breast and ovarian cancer, are passed on from both parents. As a result, in figuring out whether you may be at a higher risk for a specific disorder based on your family history, you may also want to do some homework yourself to help you and your doctor answer this first crucial question on the decision pathway.

To identify people who are at higher risk for a disorder, genetic professionals look for any one of three clues. The first (no great surprise here) is the discovery of a mutant susceptibility gene in one of the other family members. This is what happened in Todd B.'s family. It was the diagnosis of Todd's hemochromatosis that raised the red flag for other family members. He had been found to have the pair of mutations associated with this disorder showing that he had inherited one mutant gene from each of his parents. Other members of his family might also have inherited a similar genetic combination. This means that Todd's siblings, daughter, and (because the mutant gene is fairly common in some population groups) even his more distant relatives were all at a higher risk for having these same genes and for developing hemochromatosis. Although susceptibility testing is still in its early stages, many people have already used these tests to find out if they have a mutant gene that increases their susceptibility to a particular disorder. The information they have gained has been transmitted to their families in a variety of ways, ranging from an informal phone call to an announcement made at a family get-together to something even more official such as a letter. One woman agonized over how to share what she knew would be unwelcome news, and then decided to send a letter to family members. She began as follows:

> Dear Cousins,
>
> When I think of the Thompsons (and you know you're one regardless of your last name), I think about some of the things we share in varying degrees—the love of family, the love of a good time, the ability to tell a good story, the heart that's a couple sizes bigger than the bank balance, the curly hair, the freckles, and so on. Today, I am writing to let you all know of the possibility of having also inherited a mutation which is linked to an increased risk of cancer.

Whatever the means used, the message is the same: the presence of a mutant gene in one family member raises the possibility that other members of the family—male and female—may also have inherited the same flawed gene.

The second clue in determining whether someone is at a higher risk for having a flawed susceptibility gene is the presence in the family of several people with the disease, especially when that disease appears among close relatives. While there is often much interest in a family's genealogy and the tracing back of relatives through the generations, knowledge of a family's *health history* is often imperfect. However, a number of the people with whom I spoke were well aware of this health history. The disease, whichever one it was, occurred so frequently in their families that they began to believe that it was likely that they had a higher chance of coming down with it too.

> People were always sick. Since I was a child, I have been watching people die from cancer. My grandmother passed away when I was ten. She had ovarian cancer. I lost an aunt to breast cancer when I was twelve. I lost a cousin to ovarian cancer when I was sixteen. So it was always sort of around, you know, and just sort of the feeling

of watching everyone get sick and watching everyone die thinking, you know, just know . . . that obviously there is something going on.

My mother passed away at fifty-six, her mother at fifty-four, both of breast cancer. My aunt at forty-two of ovarian cancer and numerous cousins have passed away. . . . So I grew up with cancer. . . . I am not an anxiety-filled person. The fear of cancer was always in the back of my mind, but it never really affected my day-to-day living. I never really thought about it. I didn't dwell on it. But I realize now that I never saw myself as an old person. I never thought of myself as being a grandmother. I never thought of myself in old age because, to me, we didn't have that. We didn't make it out of our fifties. . . . It just didn't happen in my mind.

My uncle died of Alzheimer's, and I think he was like eighty-something, and my mother who is eighty-five has it, and my aunt who is in a nursing home is ninety-five. So, I am looking at the fact if it does hit me I am looking at being about the age of my mother. I leave my life up to God. And He has His plans for me, and if I get struck down with the disease then so be it. I will just have to do the best I can with it and my husband will do the best he can with it too.

As far as colon cancer itself, most of the members of my mother's side of the family had colon cancer at one point or another. My mother had colon cancer, and most of her brothers and sisters had it. Many of my cousins have had colon cancer. So, we assumed it was hereditary.

For others, the idea that their family may be at a higher risk for developing a disorder was not noticed at first but crept up slowly. First one person was diagnosed, and then another and, some time later, another. As one woman noted:

You know it was first the one and then the other one and then my aunts and then whoa. . . . It has made everyone a little more cautious.

For another woman, her own diagnosis of breast cancer was followed a few months later by the same diagnosis for her sister. The two events, she said, "started ringing some bells in my head." Like a puzzle whose pieces are widely scattered, when the separate pieces are finally brought together by information gathered at a family dinner, a wedding, or a funeral—piece by piece and, sometimes, over a number of years—a previously unrecognized family trend emerges. The recognition of the tendency of a certain illness to occur more often than you would expect eventually begins to take hold.

The third clue that may indicate a hereditary factor is lurking is the occurrence of a disorder—such as cancer—much earlier in a person's life than is typical. Breast cancer and ovarian cancer tend to develop after menopause. Colon cancer generally occurs after age sixty. When these illnesses occur earlier than that, it can be another red flag that may indicate that a genetic predisposition may be involved.

My father had always mentioned that his mother died young. . . . But we didn't think that much of that. When I was twenty-six, I was diagnosed with ovarian cancer, but we did not think that was family-related at the time. Then January of last year my youngest sister was diagnosed with breast cancer and went through the surgery and was going through chemo, and soon after my second-youngest sister was diagnosed with stage 3 ovarian cancer, so that is when we started thinking that this has got to be more than coincidental.

———

My mother was diagnosed with breast cancer when I was ten so I pretty much knew, had some knowledge from the time I was ten years old, that this was something that would possibly be in my future. She was thirty-four at diagnosis and thirty-seven at death. So I was pretty aware from early on and grew up very fast.

———

My mom's mom and her grandfather had already died of colon cancer by the time I was born. So, it was part of . . . the family history . . . the fact that these people were missing and had died at young ages . . . . I remember vaguely a conversation. I was sitting in the back seat of a car, and my mom was always talking about genealogy and the family history and health problems, which were basically one of the topics of car rides, and my aunt had said something about it being hereditary and genetic . . . . And so I basically have been planning for it my whole life. I have really had a hard time getting involved in any sort of relationships with people because I just sort of wonder is this person going to be a caregiver for me? Is this person strong enough actually to handle it when I get cancer at a young age?

Whether the awareness has always been there or it builds up slowly, these family narratives point to a pattern of illness that raises the possibility that something—perhaps something genetic—is going on.

Building a Family's Health History

Step One: Collecting Information

The first step, then, is to gather your own family's health history. You should do this even if you are fully convinced that your family is susceptible to a particular illness. After a health history is completed, it will be necessary to proceed to a second step: having this information evaluated by a skilled medical professional to see if there is any pattern that would point to the possible presence of a mutant susceptibility gene.

The task of putting such a family health history together can sometimes be challenging. And that process can yield important—and sometimes surprising—results.

When it comes to health care sometimes you just have to do your own leg work, you know, arm yourself with information. When I got pregnant and had my first child, I sat in the doctor's office and answered health-history questions that I had no clue about.

> Because my mother never informed me, everything was a "no."
> Does this run in your family? No. No. No. No . . . . And I am in awe
> of what I found out in the last few years that does run in my family.
> Many things that I answered "no" to should have been "yes."

A good place to begin is by consulting the family "historians," if such people already exist among your relatives. Frequently in families, there are older relatives with knowledge of several generations of family lore who may have already begun to collect information and to whom people in the family usually turn to for details about other family members. If there is no such person in your family, it will be up to you to collect and organize the family data. When sorting out all the items of information that you are collecting, either from one person or from multiple sources, it is necessary to go beyond the usual details of when people were born, married, and died. You also need to include any major medical problems that may have arisen for each person, at what age those problems first appeared, and, if it is known, the cause of death. It is important to remember that breast-cancer susceptibility genes and prostate-cancer susceptibility genes can be inherited from both male and female relatives, even though breast cancer happens mostly to women and prostate cancer happens only to men. You need to collect information about both sides of the family. Of primary interest will be the health histories of the most recent generations of your family—grandparents, parents, aunts and uncles, siblings and cousins, and that of any of your children, especially if they are adults. Though completeness is an advantage, it usually isn't necessary to track down every last individual. There is no need to trace the family tree back to the Battle of Hastings or to the Ming Dynasty. In fact, doctors consider a three-generation family history ideal.

In my previous work, I have noted the existence in some families of what I have termed a "genetic grapevine." This genetic grapevine is an informal collection of information about family health problems—and tendencies to develop health problems—that gets passed along from person to person. While this grapevine can contain useful nuggets of health data, you must be cautious. As happens in that childhood game in which you whisper something into the ear of one child who whispers it to the next child and so on, what emerges at the end can be quite different (often, in the game, hilariously so) from what was said initially. So it is with health information. What is being transmitted through the family genetic grapevine can be distorted, inaccurate, or (because such grapevines tend to persist for long periods of time) completely out of date.

Beyond drawing on the collective family memory, health information can be obtained and existing information can be verified by checking with various types of family records (that is, Bibles, personal letters, and other similar documents), consulting medical records, and obtaining death certificates. Though the rules for obtaining access to these materials differ, and access is not always possible, they can be very useful sources of information if they are available. Many people have also consulted support groups, Internet Web sites, and medical newsletters for help in explaining and decoding medical terms. A number of resources for developing and organizing your family medical history are included in the Resources section at the back of the book.

But even with the most dedicated efforts, you may not be able to collect all the information you would like. The individuals who contributed their experiences to this study pointed out some barriers that got in their way as they were trying to produce an accurate health history for their families. For example, it simply may not be possible to contact some branches of the family. Usually, when it comes to genetics, the larger the family is, the better. With more people, it is easier to discern patterns of inheritance. But large families can also present problems. The various family members can be so widely separated that they come to have limited contact with each other. One aunt and niece in this study, living at opposite ends of the country, had very different views about the extent of colon cancer in their family since each was making an assessment based solely on the cluster of relatives with whom she had contact.

Special circumstances can also intrude. Families can be so small that limited information exists. People who are adopted are often without any detailed knowledge of their biological families, let alone their health problems. Jewish individuals with families lost in the Holocaust have no way of knowing what diseases would have developed had their families been able to live out their normal lives. The sad legacy of slavery and the abuses it engendered can prevent African Americans from learning about their families or trusting the information contained in documents, such as birth certificates, which were often altered to hide the true male parent of a child. Then too, if people have drifted apart, it may be awkward to suddenly attempt contact. Sometimes, past family quarrels can also serve to permanently isolate groups of family members from one another and to make getting back in touch quite difficult.

Even when people are available and willing to share what they know, the health information they provide may be incorrect. Sometimes the medical diagnosis they received was wrong. This is particularly true for a disorder such as hemochromatosis, which can affect a number of different organs and is frequently misdiagnosed as chronic hepatitis or incorrectly attributed to the ravages of alcoholism and drug abuse. But diagnosis errors also occur for the other disorders that are serving as our model examples here. What is called liver cancer may actually have begun as colon cancer or ovarian cancer that later spread to the liver. Colon cancer and ovarian cancer are often called "irritable bowel syndrome," especially in the early stages. Alzheimer's disease is a label frequently given to any disease of the elderly that causes a deterioration in mental function even when there are other causes for that impairment.

Families may also interpret diseases in their own way. In some families, for instance, certain health subjects are taboo. Breast cancer used to be left unspoken, but that has changed recently with the frank discussion by celebrities who have successfully battled the disease and by the widespread attention given to breast-cancer awareness activities. In many places, ovarian cancer and colon cancer are still not discussed openly, or they are referred to by a "code" that makes it very hard for others to be sure of what is meant. One person was left to wonder what her grandmother actually died of. All family members would say was that "she had a cancer down there." The term "abdominal" is also used to cover—and to cover up—a multitude of health problems that people would rather not discuss. For many, mentioning the colon or talking about bowel cancer is still seen as embarrassing. In one family, "nobody said anything to anybody" about the occurrence of colon cancer. After all, as one person offered, "Who wants to talk about your colon?" Though this will change over time as it did for breast cancer, it does mean that some of the information obtained right now (about events in the past) can be incomplete or unreliable or, at best, a guess.

Although it has happened only rarely, genetic professionals have seen family situations in which incorrect information was deliberately spread. In one instance, this occurred because a grandmother didn't want people to think that there was any possibility that a flawed gene could come from her side of the family.

It is important to remember that the health history, for all its usefulness, is inevitably incomplete. The early death of individuals from accidents, war, or other causes will mean that they did not live long enough to display the symptoms of diseases such as hemochromatosis or Alzheimer's. Even if a susceptibility gene is present, breast and ovarian cancer may not show up at all in small families or in families where there may be very few women.

Just putting all the information down on paper can be a challenge. A few standard rules have been developed by geneticists to help present the information in an orderly fashion. A fictional family history, using these rules, is shown in figure 3.1. Amy (indicated by the arrow) is concerned about her half-sister Nicole (her Dad's daughter from his first marriage), who is being treated for breast cancer. Amy wants to know if she, her own daughter Chloe, and her sister Lisa are at increased risk for breast cancer. Indeed,

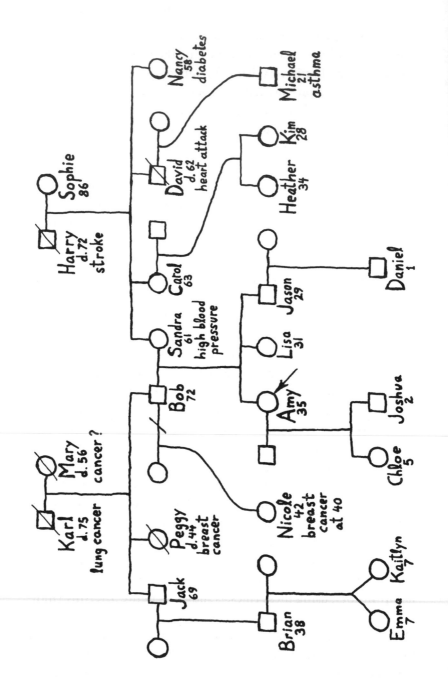

during her information-gathering process, she finds out that her Aunt Peggy died from breast cancer at age forty-four. Her grandmother Mary may also have had breast cancer, though the information here is thus far incomplete. All three female relatives diagnosed with cancer are on her Dad's side of the family. Having the health information expressed in the form of a diagram can make it easier to pick out patterns that may indicate the possible presence of mutant susceptibility genes.

Such diagrams can be drawn by hand, as shown here. But no matter how hard you try, if your Uncle Donald has had children with four different wives or your Mom's sister married your Dad's cousin, it will be hard to keep things as neat and clear as you would like. Computer software also exists to help manage the information (see Resources).

Step Two: Looking for Patterns in the Health History

After compiling your family's health history, the next step involves scrutinizing it to see whether you and your relatives may be at a higher risk for a disorder than others in the general population. Are there hints that a hereditary component may be responsible in some way for some of the illnesses that have appeared? Even with the most careful efforts at data gathering, there will be problems in identifying patterns that might point to the involvement of a flawed gene. As we saw in chapter 2 and can't repeat often enough, most common diseases are usually the result of a complex interaction

---

Figure 3.1. Diagram of a family health history. Males are shown as squares; females as circles. A slash-mark through a symbol indicates that the person has died. Parents are indicated by a horizontal line connecting their symbols; children appear below, connected to their parents by a vertical line. All the members of the same generation are shown in the same row even if there is a very large age range. Medical information (including the age when a health problem was diagnosed and/or when death occurred) is placed below the symbol for that person. Amy (indicated by the arrow) put together the diagram because of the presence of cancer in her Dad's family.

between genes and environmental factors. Some of these environmental factors can be protective, while others may accelerate the onset of a health problem. This means that some individuals who have inherited a flawed gene may never develop the disorder themselves, although they might still pass the gene along to their children. And it also means that the disorder can develop in some individuals who have no flawed gene at all. This mixture of nonhereditary and hereditary forms of the disorder—with both types able to develop in the same family—makes seeing a clear pattern difficult.

Because the identification of genetic patterns can be complicated, the best place to begin to evaluate your family health history is with your family doctor. Not to worry. Even if your doctor is not able to make an assessment from the family health history—as many are not because of their lack of training in genetics—he or she will benefit from obtaining this information and adding it to your medical record. Having this information readily available is likely to improve the medical advice that you are given in the future.

If your physician is not prepared to draw conclusions about the possible presence of a susceptibility gene in your family, it is likely that you will be referred to genetic professionals such as genetic counselors, who are experienced in doing this. Genetic professionals usually work together in groups at major medical centers. You can also locate them on your own. Check out "Ways to Find Genetic Professionals in Your Area" in the Resources section.

Genetic professionals have a number of tools at their command to make an assessment about whether you are at higher risk than what is typical in the general population:

- If a flawed susceptibility gene has already been found in one or more relatives, they can use the basic laws of inheritance and come up with an estimate of the likelihood that you too have that same flawed gene.
- If the disorder has been diagnosed in a near relative, genetic experts can provide an estimate of your risk for developing

that disorder based on what, statistically, has been observed over time for people who are close relatives of persons with that disorder. This is the type of risk figure that can be provided to the children (and other close relatives) of individuals diagnosed with Alzheimer's disease

- In some cases, they can measure the family health history you have gathered against specific criteria that have been established which indicate a heightened probability for the presence of a hereditary component. These criteria differ for each disorder. However, they all give special attention to the *number* of affected relatives (generally three or more, spanning two generations), the occurrence of the disorder in *close* relatives (parents, siblings, children), the appearance of the disorder much *earlier* than is typical (such as before age fifty for colon cancer or before menopause for breast or ovarian cancer), and *repeat* occurrences of primary tumors in one person.

- In some cases, they can use mathematical models that incorporate elements of all the approaches mentioned above and that may also incorporate other information as well (for example, findings from medical tests and pathologists' reports, or the details of one's reproductive history) to make calculations that provide an estimate of risk.

Any of these methods provides an educated guess. Because they emphasize different things, they can yield different results. In some cases, the result is an estimate of an individual's own risk for developing the disease, compared to that of the general population of the same age. For example, it may indicate that your risk is average, the same as that of the general population. Or it may indicate that your risk is considerably higher than the population risk. (Don't forget: a heightened risk can be attributed to many different nongenetic factors, as well as genetic ones.) Another method yields something quite different: an estimate of the likelihood that a flawed susceptibility gene is present in the family. For cancer, many genetics professionals recommend that genetic testing be considered if there is a 10 percent or greater probability that a mutant gene is present in the family.

No mathematical procedure can determine for certain whether or not a mutant susceptibility gene is present. Such procedures can only estimate the chance that one *may* be present. In one study, only about 60 percent of the people who fell into the high-risk category for colon-cancer susceptibility were found to have any known susceptibility genes. And susceptibility genes have been found in families that did not meet the rather stringent criteria that are used in these calculation procedures. All in all, these risk assessment tools are useful but they are only rough guides—blunt instruments, if you will.

There are also a number of risk-assessment checklists that can be found on the Internet that provide you with a risk calculation after you have answered a series of questions. Several medical centers and governmental health agencies provide tools for analyzing your personal risk of developing different types of cancer. Other checklists may be associated with commercial interests. Be careful to consider the source. Always be suspicious of a checklist that is tied in with selling specific genetic tests or other types of products.

Beware of Do-It-Yourself Risk Assessment

Even though the subject of genetics is taught in biology classes and finds its way into many media reports, most people are not skilled enough in this subject—and in the complexities of these common disorders—to be able to draw valid conclusions. In fact, when people try to make assessments on their own, a number of misconceptions and errors continually crop up. Here are some common mistakes I found.

Sometimes people drew conclusions about risk solely from the vantage point of their own family. In one family it happened, by chance, that only women had been afflicted with Alzheimer's disease. Other family members wrongly assumed that only the women in the family were at risk for the disease, not the men. In another family, one that was coping with hemochromatosis, it was wrongly assumed that only male relatives could develop the disorder. Regardless of what has been observed (especially in small families), men and women are equally likely to develop most common disorders.

Quite often, physical resemblances like eye color or skin type were taken to be sure-fire indicators that two people shared the same genes for other, more hidden, traits, like Alzheimer's or adult-onset diabetes. That's incorrect, because all of these traits are inherited independently. Having flawless skin like Aunt Betty's does not mean you have also inherited her susceptibility to colon cancer.

There is also a nearly meaningless old bit of folklore about traits "skipping a generation". This was considered to be a basic biological truth in some families, the incorrect message being that whatever shows up in the parents won't ever appear in the children but will inevitably show up in the grandchildren's generation. Typically, dominant gene mutations tend to show up in each generation. Because the involvement of other genes and of environmental factors can obscure the presence of dominant mutations in susceptibility genes, such genes can also be passed on for one or more generations without revealing themselves. There is no hard-and-fast requirement, nor is there any biological mechanism, that requires genes to reveal themselves only in alternate generations.

Since other misconceptions commonly occur, please consult with a genetic professional or knowledgeable physician before coming to any conclusion about your level of risk.

Decision Question 1: Am I at a Higher Risk than Other People?

The risk estimate that you have obtained, despite its shortcomings, is a valuable tool for helping to answer this question. However, there are other factors, besides the actual risk number itself, that can affect your answer. There is, of course, your own attitude toward risk. For some people, a 20 percent risk seems quite low; after all, this means that there is an 80 percent chance that the illness won't occur. For others, a 20 percent risk is unacceptably high. Our differing views about risk are highly personal. That's why some of us are comfortable investing in small-company stocks while others stick to bonds and money markets.

In addition, there is our own experience with particular illnesses. Medical professionals have noted that people who have taken care of someone with a serious illness—whether the ill person is a family member or a patient in the course of a work assignment—are more likely to have a deep concern about developing that illness themselves than are those who haven't had direct contact with that illness. This type of up-close and personal experience may cause specific disorders to loom large in people's minds and emotions. On the other hand, those who have seen relatives (or people they have cared for) recover well from an illness may conclude that a modest increase above the population risk is not particularly threatening. We all have our own internal gauge for what risk figure seems large—and what does not.

However you answer the question for yourself, genetic professionals and consumers agree that it is best not to make any decision about going ahead with genetic testing based just on this one factor alone. Drawing from the experiences of those who have considered genetic testing, there are three more questions you need to answer before that decision is made. We'll consider each of these questions in the next chapters.

CHAPTER FOUR

Will the Test Give Me Useful Information?

A Tale of Two Sisters

It was always clear to me that there was a pattern of cancer in my family. Five years ago my older sister, Marie, was diagnosed with breast cancer at age thirty-three. I knew at that point my sister was not interested in genetic testing. Without any evidence of a gene, or of which gene, I knew that I would have to be screened for all the mutations and the expense was going to be close to $3,000. And, even if I could afford it, I knew that if I found out one way or the other that I had a mutation then that would be information that would be very difficult for me to keep from her, and she was not ready to be tested.

Just recently, I think, once Marie got far enough out so she was feeling really good about survival, she wanted to know whether or not she had a mutant gene that would have an impact on her risk for other cancers. When I found that she was going to be tested I knew if she had a mutant gene then I would be tested. Since she was the one with the breast cancer, if she didn't have a mutant gene I wasn't going to worry so much about it anymore.

Well, Marie's test revealed the presence of a mutation in the BRCA1 gene. Armed with that information, I was tested for just that same mutation. When I went to get the results, I knew, just by looking at the genetic counselor's face when she met me in the waiting room, that I had also inherited that same mutation.

—Margaret W., age twenty-eight

Medical tests provide the data that allow conclusions to be drawn about the state of our health and, if medical problems are detected, they provide leads to the kinds of actions that may need to be taken. At first glance, nothing could seem simpler than genetic testing. After all, the only thing that is required is a sample of our genetic material, our DNA. Genetic material can easily be obtained by capturing cells from practically anywhere in the body. Procedures for analyzing DNA have been well developed, thanks to the work of genetic scientists around the world. But DNA testing for disease susceptibility turns out not to be so simple. Though genetic tests share some similarities with other medical tests, there are a number of differences associated with susceptibility-gene testing that have to be considered as you think through the value of genetic testing for yourself and your family.

What You Can—and Can't—Find Out

Many of the medical tests we take provide us with a definitive result. Yes, the urine test shows you are pregnant. Or no, the X-rays show that you have not broken a bone. Other tests can reveal whether our various body functions fall within a scale of values that is considered normal. If we are found to be too high or too low, we need to do something to correct the problem. For all the high-tech dazzle associated with the laboratory analysis in the field of susceptibility-gene testing, there is a surprising degree of uncertainty in interpreting the test results. Let's explore what can be learned—and what uncertainties persist—by looking at four common genetic testing scenarios.

Scenario One

You have had a genetic test for susceptibility to one of the four disorders being used as examples in this book. The test results are positive: you have been found to have a mutation (or, for some disorders such as hemochromatosis, a pair of mutations) that predisposes you to that disorder. The presence of the mutant gene indicates that your risk for developing the disorder is higher than that for the general population. But how much higher is it? Not all mutations are equal, and the risk figure you will be given is most likely going to be a range, say 50–85 percent by age seventy. Admittedly, we are just at the beginning of the era of genetic medicine, and medical experience with specific gene mutations is still limited. This means that the risk figure you will be given reflects the imperfect state of current medical knowledge. The number or numbers are provisional and will change as more is learned about the gene mutations themselves and the environmental factors that are involved. While having a mutant susceptibility gene raises your risk (again, by how much we cannot be sure), it is not certain that you will develop the disorder or, if you do develop it, at what age it might occur or how treatable it will be.

Scenario Two

You have a family history of breast cancer and your mother, who was treated for it several years ago, has agreed to have a genetic test to see if there might be a family mutation. Her test reveals the presence of a specific mutation in the BRCA1 gene. You go ahead now to have the DNA test—the test that looks for just that mutation—and it reveals that you do *not* have it. Here the genetic test has provided quite useful information. You are, in the jargon of the field, a "true negative." Because you have not inherited the family mutation, you are no longer considered to be at higher risk than other people. Keep in mind that many different genes and environmental factors interact in complicated and poorly understood ways to bring on most common illnesses, including breast cancer. Therefore, the absence of the mutant gene does not guarantee that you will be spared the disorder during your lifetime. However, your risk of developing the disorder is now only average. It is no greater than it is for people in the general population.

Scenario Three

You are the first person in your family being tested for a susceptibility mutation for colon cancer. When you receive your genetic test result, it says that you do *not* have any known mutation. Here the finding that no known mutation is present is less reassuring than it was in Scenario Two. It is always possible that another, still undiscovered, mutant susceptibility gene may be circulating in your family. As Susan Tinley, genetic nurse at Creighton University, explains, "I think it is so important for people to be aware that when we are doing that first test in the family, if that result comes back negative, it's not a true negative. There are limitations in terms of the capability of this testing so that if that first test in the family comes back negative, you haven't completely ruled out the presence of a mutation because there may be some types of mutations within a known susceptibility gene that we cannot detect, or there may be other genes that have not been identified yet."

Scenario Four

Your test results come back and show that there is a variation— one that has not been seen before—in the DNA of one of the susceptibility genes that were examined. However, it is not known if this particular change in the DNA is just a neutral variation, the type that occurs frequently in DNA and is without any effect on your future health, or if it is a variation that raises your chances of illness. In such a situation, you will be told that you possess a "genetic variant of unknown significance" or a "genetic variant of uncertain clinical significance." In colon cancer and breast-cancer susceptibility testing, this happens about 10 percent of the time. Future research on this variation will reveal whether it increases risk appreciably, only slightly, or not at all. But for the moment, no one knows what, if anything, it means.

These four scenarios demonstrate that genetic tests for disease susceptibility seldom offer an easy "yes" or "no" answer. In fact, it can often be difficult to draw firm conclusions. The presence of a mutation is not a harbinger of inevitable illness, and the absence of a mutation is not assurance of freedom from illness. The bottom line is that both the person seeking useful and meaningful results and the medical professional attempting to interpret the results confront uncertainties and often must struggle to extract meaning from the probability figures or range of percentages that invariably accompany susceptibility-gene testing.

The Importance of Knowing Just What You Are Looking For

Medical tests typically involve only the person being tested. Many of the original genetic tests—the prenatal tests and the carrier tests that launched the genetic revolution in medicine are similar in that only the individual about whom the information is sought needs to be tested. However, when it comes to susceptibility-gene testing, it may be that someone else—another family member—has to be tested first.

When an increased susceptibility to a particular disorder can be brought on by any one of a large number of different mutations in any of several genes, as is the case with breast cancer and colon cancer, then genetic testing should ideally be done in two stages The first stage requires the testing of a person in the family who has already been diagnosed with the disorder. This is the person who is most likely to reveal whether a genetic flaw is actually present—and which one it is. In the case of Margaret W.'s family, learning that Marie had a flawed gene permitted Margaret (and other family members as well) to be examined for that same flaw. Those family members who do not have that same genetic flaw are the "true negatives" that we spoke of in Scenario Two. Those who are found to have inherited that flaw, as Margaret did, now know that they are at an increased risk for breast/ovarian cancer.

Beginning the testing process with a relative who has had the disorder allows the specific genetic flaw, if present, to be recognized and to be searched for in other family members. This procedure can be likened to the use of wanted posters in the old days of the Wild West. The marshal needed that poster in order to know what the bad guy looked like so that he could pick him out from the crowd of similarly dressed patrons in the saloon. Without the benefit of the poster, the marshal would not know whether the bad guy was right there or had never been in town at all.

Of course, if that first test of a person in the family with the disorder comes back negative (no known mutation is found), you haven't completely ruled out the presence of a mutation because, as in Scenario Three, there may still be undetected mutations within the known susceptibility genes or there may be mutations hiding in other susceptibility genes that have not yet been identified.

The main requirement for this two-stage testing process to unfold properly is that someone in the family who has the illness— or who had once had it—has to agree to be tested first. Genetic professionals say that it is rare for the person with the illness to refuse to participate in the initial stage of the testing process if he or she has been asked to do so by another family member. But consumers report that this need to first test another person can produce complications. Sometimes, there are simply no survivors to ask and no access to their tissue samples. Or the family may have grown so distant—not only geographically but also as a result of discord or lack of communication—that it can be extremely awkward, if not impossible, to get in touch and to make the request. And sometimes the family member may be alive and approachable but not willing to undergo the test. For example:

> Well, I knew that nobody in my family was interested in testing because we had had conversations before that. They weren't interested in the test at all, and I knew it. . . . I think it was a fear factor. And you know . . . I could have imposed upon my mother and could have really made her do it. She would have done it if I would have begged her to do it, but it would have caused her so much anxiety and it would have been really problematic. She was scared of it. And I am telling this as part of the story because I think it's really a problem. And I know a lot of people that haven't taken the test or it took them an extra year because they had to deal with their family members or they had to dig up old tissue samples from dead relatives.

The resistance of others in the family to helping you can be troubling. It is important to keep in mind that no matter how much you want them to do it, their personal decision not to be tested is one that has to be respected because every individual has the right to decide what is done to his or her body.

This two-stage testing process is likely to become even more necessary in the future as additional susceptibility genes for common illnesses are found and as a large number of possible mutations in those genes are identified.

Considering the Costs of the Testing

As with any type of testing, paying for it can be an issue. For those who have been referred to, or who have gotten themselves to, a unit or department specializing in medical genetics, there will first be the cost of the genetic counseling that is standard. The cost of the counseling session is usually modest, especially when one considers that this visit can take an hour or more. Often, genetic counseling appointments are covered as office visits under insurance plans. But this cost should be factored in as you consider whether susceptibility testing is affordable.

The costs of the genetic testing itself can range widely, from a few hundred dollars for the mutations associated with hereditary hemochromatosis or Alzheimer's disease to thousands of dollars for susceptibility-gene mutations associated with cancer. For each type of testing, costs are lower if the specific mutation in the family has already been determined, since it is now only necessary to test for one specific mutation rather than searching for all possible ones. Testing costs can also be lower if the individual belongs to an ethnic group in which only a few mutations are prevalent. Thus, breast/ovarian cancer susceptibility-gene testing in Jewish families of European (Ashkenazi) ancestry can focus on the three major mutations that occur most frequently in this group, rather than on a larger number of mutations.

Costs can vary based on how the tests are done and whether additional, nongenetic, tests are included. Insurance companies, Medicare, and Medicaid have different policies about payment for genetic tests. It will be necessary to contact your provider to determine what the coverage is and what portion, if anything, you will be expected to pay. Copayments can sometimes be steep. Large genetic-testing laboratories check on the level of insurance coverage and make sure that people are "preauthorized" by the insurance company to avoid later problems in payment.

For people without health insurance, the costs of testing can put it out of reach. Said one woman after a diagnosis of hemochromatosis in her family:

> It's very expensive, and we cannot afford it. My one brother has only seasonal work. His daughters live with his ex-wife, and he can't afford to send money for them to be tested as well. So, right now, it really is the money factor because it is so expensive. I think they would all go and have testing if it wasn't for the fact of the money needed.

The extra cost associated with testing another person, in the two-stage testing process, may also be an issue. Since it is highly unlikely that an insurance company would pay the costs of testing someone they do not cover, the first person being tested, whether it is Cousin Sadie or Uncle Rocco, must pay for it themselves or through their own insurance carriers. In a few cases, the family member who requested the testing of a relative has paid for that relative's test. There have been times when groups of family members pitched in and collected money to help subsidize the costs of testing that first relative.

Because of concerns about insurance discrimination if a genetic mutation is found, some people in this study who had health insurance nevertheless opted to pay the full costs themselves to keep their testing under the radar of the insurance company. We will look further into these concerns in chapter 6.

The Personal Impacts of Genetic Testing

Many medical tests bring along more with them than just the test results. There can be anxiety while waiting to hear the outcome as well as emotionally painful reactions to the results themselves.

Susceptibility-gene testing can evoke similar reactions, and these reactions may even be intensified because of the special status that has been accorded genes in current-day society. Psychological distress can occur at many points during the testing process.

The time interval between sending a DNA sample for testing and getting the results back can be from one to several weeks. During this waiting period, the reactions reported by the consumers consulted in this study ranged from minor concern to major apprehension, but, generally, they were not much different from what people experience while waiting for the results of other types of major medical tests:

> It was more of a curiosity because, honestly, I felt like it was probably going to be positive. So it was more of a hope it might be negative that was in my mind, but it wasn't something that I stressed about every day.

> I was anxious about it, you know, kind of concerned about seeing what my sister has gone through and not wanting to go through some of the same things she is having to endure.

> I careened back and forth from assuming the best to fearing the worst.

The results can be reported back in several different ways: face-to-face during a planned office visit, by phone, in the mail, or through e-mail. Since the advent of genetic testing in the closing decades of the twentieth century, genetic professionals as well as individuals who have undergone genetic testing have noted that the response to receiving the test results can be unexpectedly powerful and distressing. Susceptibility-gene testing is no different.

Some consumers interviewed for this study took the report of a positive result—the finding that a mutation was present in a susceptibility gene—quite calmly. One woman, who had just learned of a BRCA1 mutation, went out to a movie to let the information sink in. Another woman was equally unruffled:

> I was remarkably not surprised and the genetic counselor commented that I didn't appear to be surprised. Given the 50/50 nature of it, I had figured that this was a high likelihood I had it, and so I had chosen to look at it that way. And I tend to be an optimist, but for some reason I really saw this as a highly likely event.

There was even a degree of comfort:

> I felt relieved to know what my mother, my aunt, and my grandmother didn't know. They never knew what hit them. So for me it kind of solved the family mystery. I was really devastated for a day and then I just recovered from it and decided, in my own mindset, that it was good knowledge to have, and I am really lucky to be able to find out my own status.

Others, too, have indicated that they were grateful to find from the test that the "smoking gun" in the family was a flaw in a gene. Now the family finger-pointers looking to assign blame could be told it was a gene and was not, as had been whispered about in some families, their drinking habits, or diet, or, as one young woman put it, their "really bad karma."

However, even when positive results were expected, actually hearing that the genetic test has verified the presence of a mutation can produce unexpectedly strong and unpleasant reactions. For some, it was like an emotional earthquake. One volunteer, associated with a patient support group, has seen these reactions many times:

> I will get calls where the person is crying and they can't even talk. So, my automatic response is: You have got your test back and it was positive, right?

When a mutation is found that predisposes people to future illness, many people do struggle with shock, depression, and anger.

When I went back to get the test results, I didn't even take my husband with me. I didn't think I was going to have it. I really lacked the cancer history that makes some people so sure they have it. And this very nice woman says we have your results and they are positive, and I go, "Oh shit." I didn't cry or break down or any thing, but I was just kind of numb. Then I came home and cried, you know, just kind of lost it.

———

It was a week of my husband and me crying because we had just gone through so much dealing with my own cancer. You think you are done with everything and then it's an immediate whammy. And there is no support. There was no support in the community. Nobody knew how to talk to you. You are very isolated with this information. And it's great to have the information, but you are kind of tossed back out there on the street with it, which was incredibly hard to manage.

———

I thought I was absolutely ready. I expected to be positive and I thought well, you know, this obviously wasn't going to affect me because I already had cancer and then the report came back that it was positive, and I found myself emotionally just overwhelmed. And I cried as if I had never known anything. So that was a big shock to me, my reaction to it. I definitely became depressed and sad over the whole thing.

———

When I first found out, I thought about it 24/7. Am I going to get the cancer? When am I going to get it? What will happen if I get the cancer? How old will the kids be? Will my husband remarry? I mean I know it sounds crazy, but those thoughts went through my head all the time. There is not a day that goes by that I don't think about it. It's been a year now so some days are better than others. I don't think about it quite as much. And I have realized that whatever happens, happens.

Even though geneticists know that each and every one of us carries some ten flaws in our DNA, the fact that a genetic test can find one of those previously hypothetical mutations and assign a particular genetic label to you has left many people feeling diminished and frightened.

In contrast, one would think that a negative result—that is, the genetic test does not find any known mutation—would generate relief. But here too, the reality is a lot more complex. For those who were found to be "true negatives" as in Scenario Two—they did not inherit the family mutation—there was certainly much relief and even, for one man, euphoria. But sometimes there was a price. And that price goes by the term "survivor guilt." Survivor guilt has long been noted in life-and-death situations—wars, natural disasters, traffic accidents, and the like—in which some people manage to stay alive while others die. Often those who survive such situations are left to wrestle with feelings of guilt about why they were spared while others, just like themselves, were not. Genetic professionals have long been aware that genetic test results can bring on survivor guilt when some family members inherit a particular mutation and others do not. Susceptibility-gene testing is no different in this regard. In one case, the survivor guilt appeared from the very moment that siblings got their genetic-test results. Here is the counselor's recollection:

> I had three siblings who came in for their results together and two of the three were positive for the mutation. The two that were positive for the mutation, they were very upbeat after they got the results, almost as if they were expecting it to happen. The one that really looked sad was the one that didn't have it. The two that were positive were trying to comfort him. I remember one of them saying, "We always thought you were the milkman's baby."

Survivor guilt can emerge later, after knowledge of the test results sinks in. One woman, with a known mutation, described her brother's reaction when he found out that he did not inherit the family's predisposition to colon cancer.

> He was elated. He was. He truly was. He left a message on my phone, and he was just bubbling. Oh, what a relief! Oh my god, he

was so glad he had done it now, and he was so glad to have the results, and it meant he didn't have to have this conversation with his daughters further down the road. And then, he must have thought of me. He just stopped and caught his breath, and he said, "Oh my gosh, I feel kind of guilty." But I called him right back and told him that is ridiculous. He shouldn't be feeling guilty. I am extremely happy for him. I really am.

There are many manifestations of this phenomenon. Survivor guilt can also be borne in silence when family members who have tested negative for the family mutation choose to keep that information from their mutation-positive siblings. Or people have given incorrect information about their genetic test results to their families so that they would fit in with the others or diminish their concerns. And sometimes the emotional tugs of survivor guilt can operate in reverse. One woman, found to have a BRCA1 mutation, came to feel (not unreasonably) that because of all the risk-reduction actions she had taken, she was now at a lower risk of developing breast cancer than her sister who did not have the mutant gene. So she began to experience survivor guilt herself. However and whenever it arises, genetic counselors urge their clients to be careful that survivor guilt is dealt with openly, so that it doesn't become a wedge separating people in the family from one another.

Unlike the true negatives—those who have escaped the family mutation—the individuals who receive a negative test result when their family mutation is not known (as in Scenario Three above) can be angry and upset. Their search for definitive information has been unsuccessful. For example:

I am bummed out. I really am, I am disappointed. . . . I just feel kind of like a sitting duck.

_____

I don't believe that the negative test completely relieved my mind. It is bittersweet since you don't know what mutation you are looking for and the legacy of cancer is still there.

_____

> Do you go and test again and again [as more susceptibility genes are found]? Do you upgrade [the test] like you do your Windows software?

————

> I had mixed feelings, to tell the truth. I thought I would be ecstatic, but in some ways it made both my decision-making process about treatment more difficult, and it also put me in a sort of great unknown as far as the risks of my other family members and my future risks of cancers, because I still think that there is something in my family.

For these folks, a negative result from the genetic testing process did not provide any firm information beyond what they already knew prior to the test. They are left to struggle with a number of questions: What is their real risk? What is the explanation for the illness that they feel is so strikingly prevalent in their families? Is it possible that they have a mutation in an unknown gene, one that has not yet been identified by the researchers? What is the best way to protect their own health? Should they be tested continually for mutations in each new susceptibility gene that medical research discovers? The reality is that until research yields complete information about the full array of genes involved in the disease, answers to these questions will be slow in coming.

Those whose susceptibility-test results indicate that there is a "variant of unknown significance" (as in Scenario Four) are frequently left frustrated, suspended between worry and relief.

> Well, I was disappointed. I just kind of said, "Okay, so what does that mean?" And they went through more statistics, and I was very emotional, I was very disappointed. I didn't start getting super emotional, I didn't cry or anything until she started talking about my kids because that is the big thing for me—are they going to be potentially affected?

As one genetic counselor reports, "You are essentially saying—well, we found something we really can't explain. Chances are it's harmless, but we can't really tell you that with any certainty. And once we said that, it's really hard to dislodge that idea they get in their minds that there is something there and they are really in a quandary over what to do about it." Over time, as researchers learn more about these variants and whether or not they are correlated with the onset of disorders, it should be possible to come away with more certain information. However, few effective pathways exist thus far to recontact and inform individuals years down the road, when this information emerges.

As we have seen here, regardless of the testing scenario, susceptibility-gene testing can evoke strong reactions, and there can be significant emotional fallout from the test results that are received. While such reactions may not be of long duration or be sufficiently compelling to either go ahead with testing or to decline it, it is important to consider the kinds of effects that you may experience—or which might arise in your family—and to take them into account as part of the decision process.

Informing the Family

When we are sitting around the Thanksgiving table with our family, enjoying the wonderfully delicious, cholesterol-laden cuisine, the subject of our cholesterol numbers can come up. In that friendly atmosphere, our test results—and maybe what medications we are taking when those numbers are too high—may be shared. But usually we are not eager to distribute our own medical details too widely. Such information is generally kept close to home, or is confined to the special relationship that exists between physician and patient and the cloak of confidentiality that is central to that relationship.

Because of the importance accorded to genes in our society, and the all-too-often—and unfortunate—stigma associated with having a known genetic flaw, genetic information tends to be especially closely guarded. Many consumers have taken steps themselves to make sure that their health insurance companies don't find out that a test has been done. And many states in the United States have dealt with the need for genetic privacy through laws and policies designed to protect people from the harm that could occur if genetic data are released.

But, as we saw in chapter 1, genetic information is also different from other medical information because genes are shared within families. If one person in a family has been tested and is found to have a mutant susceptibility gene, it is likely that others in the family have inherited that same flawed gene. In this situation, it is generally held that family members should know about their possibility of having inherited such a mutant gene, particularly if this information could be of use in their immediate health decisions. You cannot count on relatives learning of their heightened risk independently either from their own doctors or by figuring it out on their own. And you cannot count on your doctor to inform family members. In fact, it's frowned on by traditional medical ethics and prohibited by the more recent Health Insurance Portability and Accountability Act (HIPAA). So it's up to you. Sharing your genetic information with your own family is not a legal requirement. However, it is generally considered to be a morally worthy thing, within families, to look out for one another's well-being. This translates to a responsibility to inform other people in the family of a positive genetic-test result, so that they will be aware that they may be at a higher risk for a particular illness. How your relatives choose to use this information is, of course, up to them. They must make their own decisions. Several of the consumers in this study did not consider the sharing of their own genetic information an onerous task but rather felt it was a "gift" that they gladly gave to their relatives.

Actually delivering this information can be hard to do. Various modes of contact are used. The phoning of close relatives is the most common. Broaching the possibility of a genetic flaw residing in members of the immediate family—parents, siblings, adult children (we'll get to younger children in the next chapter)—is never an easy matter. Explanations involve the concepts and vocabulary of genetics. These can be difficult to express, especially if you are struggling with that information yourself. It is important to be sure that your test result is not misunderstood. People should not be left thinking that the onset of an illness is inevitable. If the testing was carried out under the auspices of a genetic-counseling program, genetic counselors will be able to assist you by providing a letter explaining the situation to family members, in user-friendly language. The letter can also include information describing the test or tests that are available.

All families are different and reactions to the information will vary. One reaction that arises in all types of susceptibility-gene testing (as it does in other types of genetic testing) is that of "parental guilt." Even though we receive our genes by chance and pass them along to our children, again by chance, some parents still feel that they are personally at fault for passing along a susceptibility mutation that puts their children at increased risk. One father, for example, was stricken at the thought that he was a carrier of a mutant BRCA1 gene and that he had passed that gene on to his daughters:

> He was really sad. He was sad. It wasn't his own mortality, it wasn't the fact that he could be at risk, but he was undone at the thought that he has passed this on to his daughters. I think that he just felt a certain amount of guilt. I told him there's nothing, obviously, there is nothing that you should, could, have done to prevent it short of not having children. And he said to me that he would never have traded any of us for knowing he hadn't passed on that kind of thing. So, that sort of gave him some comfort, but I think at the same time he felt it was one of those things that, as a parent, you don't want your child to have to carry that.

One woman's feelings of guilt and shame led her to secretly wish that she could assign blame to her husband:

> Well, to be honest this sounds terrible, but you know I was thinking to myself it would be really nice if something was wrong with him, and I am not the one that gave it to my kids, but he didn't have anything.

Even more difficult than conveying genetic information within the immediate family is attempting to expand the zone of contact to reach out to more far-flung branches of the family—aunts, uncles, and cousins. Family letters are used (we saw a small sample on page 24), as well as announcements at occasions when the family gets together. For some, it can feel like being thrust into the role of the Ancient Mariner of the Coleridge poem who collars passing strangers to share his tale of woe. One genetic counselor, cognizant of the discomfort that can arise on both sides in such conversations, suggests that people should say by phone or by mail something like: "I have had genetic counseling and testing. If you would like further information about my experience or what was found, I am happy to share it with you." This gives relatives the opportunity to ask for more information or to decline interest. At the same time, it keeps the door open for them to get back in touch for the information in the future. Depending on the family dynamics, the responses can vary from gratitude for the information to denial ("This doesn't apply to me"). One man, sharing news about hereditary hemochromatosis with relatives, referred to one type of reaction as smugness ("You're not going to pin this on me. It may be in your branch of the family, but it's not in mine").

Many people have made valiant efforts to reach the relatives who might be at risk. On occasion it meant trusting that family members would pass the information along. "It went through a chain of hands," said one woman, "and I don't know how well the information got relayed." For some, it meant finding ways around relatives who were bottlenecks in the information-transfer process—and many families seem to have such relatives—in order to inform their children who might be at risk. It is a very imperfect process. Sadly, a few individuals interviewed in this study were unable to embark on this family mission to share their genetic findings because of lost contact over the years, emotional residue from past family bitterness, and personal pain (from the knowledge of their own genetic status) that prevented them from sharing their genetic information with anyone.

Selecting the Right Genetic Testing Venue

Currently, genetic tests can be obtained in several different types of settings. Genetic tests for susceptibility can be ordered by your own physician, just as other medical tests are. In this type of arrangement, there is the value of the physician's close knowledge of your medical history and personal preferences. There is also the opportunity for careful and ongoing attention after the test results are received. Keep in mind that these are still the early days of genetic medicine. Many physicians have not yet had sufficient training in genetics and, despite their best efforts, they may have difficulty interpreting the genetic-test results. Physicians do tend to be directive in their advice and their strong preferences are valued when choices need to be made among different medical treatments. However, when it comes to genetic testing their strong preferences can get in the way of making your own personal decision. Then too, the hectic environment of a busy medical office may allow little time for educating patients and answering their questions about genetic matters.

Tests can also be arranged at genetics centers where a variety of genetic services are offered. Such centers are generally found in major teaching hospitals or as part of a clinic with a focus on a particular disorder such as colon cancer or breast cancer. This type of specialty center offers access to a team of genetic professionals, including genetic counselors. Figure 4.1 shows a genetic counselor working with clients during a genetic counseling session. Genetic counselors can help obtain medical records, evaluate the family history, explain scientific information, provide informed interpretation of test results, and, in many places, they can help deal with any psychological or other after-effects of the test. Spouses, other family members, and even good friends can be included at any of the meetings if the client wishes. Genetic professionals at these centers or clinics attempt to be nondirective in their approach. This means that they neither promote nor discourage testing, but instead seek to assist their clients as their clients make their own

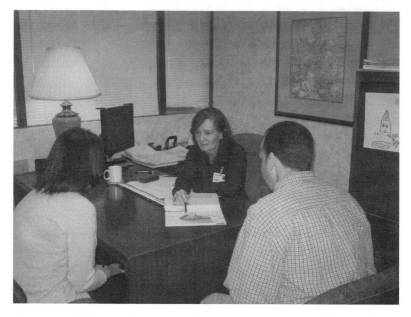

Figure 4.1. A photograph of a genetic counseling session. Genetic counselors meet with their clients to discuss a broad range of health issues
related to genetics. Genetic testing options are only one of many issues
that can be pursued in such sessions.

decisions. However, genetic counseling units may not always be
conveniently located. Travel to them from outlying areas can be a
problem, especially when several visits need to be made.

There is a third possibility: arranging genetic tests through private laboratories that deal directly with the consumer by advertis-
ing their services in magazines, on television, and on the Internet.
With this approach, there can be savings in time and effort:

> If you go down to the city to where they do the counseling and the
> breast-cancer gene testing, you have to go once for a family history
> and counseling. You have to make a second trip down to do the
> blood draw and you have to make a third trip down to be given the
> test results face-to-face. I chose to bypass the way most do it

because I just felt like they were making me jump through more hoops than I needed to and it meant three days I was going to have to take a day out of my life and drive to the city and arrange child care. I just found a way to bypass that.

In this third genetic-testing mode, the consumer is operating independently of the usual medical channels. The different companies operating in this mode follow a variety of practices. As a result, consumers can get different degrees of information and assistance prior to testing and after the results come in. There are concerns, of course, that since the companies' financial well-being is connected with payment for the tests, these organizations may not be able to provide enough opportunity for choice beforehand and they may be too impersonal, offering only a limited support system afterward if that should be needed. Of those interviewed for this study who had worked through a professional genetic-services center, there was skepticism about striking off on your own for genetic information and testing.

I consider myself fairly educated about breast cancer and somewhat about genetics, but I did not know until I went through that process that, yes, I could get a negative result, but it wouldn't really change anything for me. So I have real problems with the thought of someone having testing and not going through the process, the educational process, they need to have and the support they need to have.

———

Somebody has to deal with the emotional side of it, and it's not just about taking the test. Taking the test is really the easy part, you know. It's a relatively simple test. It's the emotional aspect that's hard. What are you going to do if, what if?

Only about half of the people in this study who opted for genetic testing had any form of genetic counseling prior to the testing. As the field of genetic medicine matures and the number of susceptibility tests increases, it is likely that other novel means of delivery of genetic services will be developed. It is vital that consumers select the venues in which they will be given the best evaluation of their family history, the fullest chance to learn and to ask questions, the freedom to make their own decisions without subtle or not-so-subtle coercion, and the opportunity to establish personal plans of action to improve their long-term health, regardless of what testing decision is made.

Decision Question 2: Will the Genetic Test Give Me Useful Information?

This question is a crucial component of the decision process. It is a complicated question because there are so many aspects to consider. These include:

- any pre-test requirements, especially if it is necessary for someone else in your family—someone who has already had the illness—to be tested first to find out if there is a family mutation;
- your understanding of possible test outcomes: a positive result (showing an increase in risk ranging from very large to quite small, depending on the mutation), a negative result (showing no increase over average risk), and an indeterminate result;
- the cost of testing;
- how you will deal with any emotional reactions that may accompany the test;
- the ways you will share, with your immediate and more-extended family, a test result that shows the presence of a mutant gene.

Overall, you must determine if the test procedures can yield a result that will be meaningful to you. You must also examine the environment within which susceptibility-gene testing would be carried out in order to be sure that the necessary components of susceptibility testing—risk assessment, education, choice, interpretation, and support—are suited to your needs.

Once you have answered this question, you are well on your way to making your genetic-testing decision. But you are not done yet. There are still two more questions that you need to consider. Keep reading!

CHAPTER FIVE

Is This the Right Time in My Life to Be Taking This Test?

Waiting Gloom

When I was a little girl, we took care of my grandmother while she was sick with ovarian cancer. When my mother was diagnosed with the same thing, my immediate thought was that this is a death sentence and there's nothing I can do about it. After my mother's surgery, the doctor came out and explained to us that she had ovarian cancer and then he looked straight at me and said, "I would highly recommend genetic testing for you at this point." I contacted the genetic counselor but I have not been tested yet, and it's been one of those things hanging over my head for the last two years. My children are young and they need me. I help my husband run his business. When things settle down with my mother, I would like to have the testing done. At first she did not want to be tested but finally a couple of months ago she said she might be willing to be tested. Right now, though, she's dealing with the chemotherapy and the whole state of life at the moment and she doesn't want anything to do with it.

I suppose I could go ahead and be tested without waiting for my mother's results. There is only so much I can afford to have hanging at once. My life is not in the place where I could take that on. I think that is part of the reason I haven't done it yet. But I believe that the biggest—and most honest—reason that I haven't tested yet is that I am afraid that a positive result would send my mother into such a deep depression that she would lose her desire to fight.

—Carmela C., age thirty-four

In some medical situations, timing is crucial. Familiar images from TV medical dramas portray patients rushed into surgery and show teams of doctors and nurses hurrying to bedsides to restart hearts or administer life-saving medication—all without a second to spare. Moments of such urgency seldom occur in susceptibility gene testing. This type of gene testing can usually proceed without the pressure of time. Nonetheless, time—or, better, timing—is a key element that must be factored into any testing decision.

Realistically, it is always best to make genetic-test decisions (and, of course, any other important decisions) when one's life is in a calm place. One person in this study put it this way:

At certain points in your life you are ready to hear this information. Other times, no—if other things are going on.

This view is seconded by genetic counselor Gladys Rosenthal: "I think that if you're living a stressful life trying to make ends meet, if you have got a lot of other things going on in your life, or if you are meeting one crisis after another, then I don't think that is the time to be looking for things that might happen in the future." As a general rule, then, periods in one's life that are rife with painful transitions—divorce, death, job loss—or burdened with over-whelming responsibilities—whether those be in the family, at school, or at work—are not the best moments to confront the additional intellectual and emotional demands of genetic testing.

There are two specific timing issues that do enter into susceptibility-gene testing. First, people seeking testing may not be able to proceed until the cooperation of other family members is obtained. Second, children may have to wait until they reach adulthood before getting tested.

Family Cooperation

As we have seen in chapter 4, if several different mutations in susceptibility genes are implicated in the development of a disorder (as in breast cancer, for example), it is important to test a family member who has been diagnosed with the disorder to see if a known mutation is present. Family members are often willing to cooperate and, if a mutation is found, you and anyone else in the family can be tested for just that particular mutation.

Even though the family member you have approached is willing to help, it may happen that the time is not right for that relative to have genetic testing. Consumers reported a variety of delays that cropped up. Prominent among these were the family member's own medical struggle with the illness, especially if that person was in the process of undergoing treatments that were invasive or exhausting. This, as we have seen in the interview extract above, was the situation for Carmela C. Her mother was in too precarious a physical and emotional state for genetic testing to be done. Others have faced problems when relatives were distracted by highly stressful events in their lives, or, for reasons of age and advanced illness, were no longer mentally competent and thus unable to consent for themselves.

For various reasons, then, undergoing susceptibility-gene testing on behalf of even a much-loved relative (in order to see if there is a family mutation) can be given low priority. Later on, the situation may change. However, one can never be sure just how long it will be until that happens. On occasion, it may be possible to speed up matters by arranging for the testing of samples (if these are available) from tissues that were removed during surgery and then archived in pathology laboratories. But tracking those samples down and getting permission to use them will also take effort—and, yes, time.

Stage of Life

There are periods in a person's life when it may not be appropriate to carry out susceptibility testing. For most of the disorders where susceptibility genes can be involved, the first symptoms appear in the adult years. This raises the issue about whether youngsters should be tested to see if they've inherited susceptibility genes found in their parents, when the effects of such genes may not be revealed for decades, if at all. As an example, should teenage girls be tested for the presence of a BRCA1 or BRCA2 gene mutation found in their families? Some parents believe that it is their right to decide, on behalf of their children, whether genetic testing should be carried out—just as they decide on other medical matters. However, the general consensus within the community of genetic professionals is that these are situations in which such testing of otherwise-healthy children should *not* be done. They offer two main concerns that give rise to this view.

The first concern is that the harm of knowing about a genetic mutation at a young age may exceed any benefit that could be gained. If there are no actions that can be taken early in life to prevent (or reduce the chance of) the later onset of illness associated with the mutation, or to reduce the severity of the later illness, there is no benefit for the child to have this information. Not only would this knowledge not be helpful, it could be harmful. It is possible that the child could feel stigmatized and suffer psychological injury from this information. Even if he or she is not told the test results (or doesn't understand them), harm could result if parents or siblings treat the child differently because of their knowledge of the genetic situation. Harm could also result if that information finds its way to third parties such as teachers or classmates. If there is no health benefit to be gained by knowing early in life, then there would seem to be no reason to test and to run the risk of these problems.

The second concern about susceptibility testing early in life draws on lessons learned by genetic professionals with previous forms of DNA testing, particularly the testing for Huntington disease. Huntington is a disorder that appears in the middle decades of life for those who have inherited a single mutant gene. It is marked by severe neurological and psychiatric symptoms that ultimately lead to death. There is no cure at present. Even though a test for the mutant gene is available, about 80 percent of adults who have a parent with Huntington (and who thus have a 50/50 chance of developing it themselves) have decided against taking this test. Decisions by consumers to forgo the newer susceptibility-gene tests are also evidence that people do not always want to have genetic information. The testing of young children for disorders that occur much later in life denies those children the chance to make that same decision when they are older. Genetic susceptibility testing is, therefore, best deferred to the adult years when the children at risk have grown up and can now make up their own minds to opt for it or against it.

Professional organizations have put forth policies that advocate waiting until the child is old enough to decide, usually at eighteen years of age or older. The American Medical Association has, as part of its guidelines on the genetic testing of children, the following statement:

> When a child is at risk for a genetic condition with adult onset for which preventive or other therapeutic measures are not available, genetic testing of children generally should not be undertaken. Families should still be informed of the existence of tests and given the opportunity to discuss the reasons why the tests are generally not offered for children.

The American Society of Human Genetics and the American College of Medical Genetics, whose members are genetic professionals, have issued a joint statement in accord with this: "If the medical or psychosocial benefits of a genetic test will not accrue until adulthood, as in the case of . . . adult-onset diseases, genetic testing generally should be deferred." Other advisory bodies in the U.S. and internationally that have been convened to consider the issue of genetic testing of children have also endorsed this position.

Special circumstances can arise which even the most thorough of guidelines cannot anticipate. For example, a young teen, fully capable of evaluating the pros and cons of susceptibility testing, may request testing because of severe anxieties connected to her experiences with the disorder as it developed in her family. Or an adolescent may be sexually active and there is the prospect that a potential pregnancy would put another individual at risk. The details of these exceptions will differ. However they arise, it is important to remember that the main consideration is the well being of the child, not the fears, unease, or passing interests of the parents or of anyone else, for that matter. And if such testing is done, special efforts should be made to ensure that the setting and the procedures are comfortable for the child involved. What is suitable for the genetic testing of an adult may not be so for a child.

This general prohibition on genetic testing of children for their susceptibility to late-onset disorders evaporates if early knowledge of genetic status could provide some clear benefit. This benefit could be in the form of diet or medications known to thwart the onset of the illness. Or it could be in the form of close monitoring during childhood to enable early detection of the start of the disease and the initiation of treatments that are most effective when started promptly. Current examples of situations in which genetic testing is appropriate include multiple endocrine neoplasia (MEN), Factor V Leiden clotting disorder, and familial adenomatous polyposis (FAP).

For hereditary hemochromatosis, there is some disagreement about whether genetic testing meets the standard for testing in childhood. Some groups in favor of hemochromatosis genetic testing at an early age argue that caution with diet (such as avoiding iron-enriched cereals) and early detection of high iron levels in the blood are valuable health benefits that justify such testing. Other groups hold that organ damage seldom occurs before adulthood so that decisions on genetic testing could be deferred until then.

Not surprisingly, the parents in this study were of various minds when it came to susceptibility testing for their children. Most agreed that testing too early carried with it the possibility of problems, such as emotional distress, without any compensating benefits. For breast/ovarian cancer and colon-cancer susceptibility, most parents felt that the earliest any genetic testing for susceptibility should be done was the late teens or early twenties. The testing of children for susceptibility to the classic late-onset form of Alzheimer's disease was widely rejected. However, in families at risk for hemochromatosis, the parents were as divided as the medical community about the merits of testing their children. Several families had gone ahead to test their children for the known susceptibility genes; others had chosen not to test.

> Well, she was seven when we found out she had both genes. The doctors really don't even know what they are really looking at when it comes to the iron ranges of children because it's not really anything that has been explored in great depth. But anyway, the pediatrician said that she didn't think it was a concern at this point.
>
> ———
>
> My six-year-old was tested a month after I had myself tested. It was within weeks probably, I can't remember exactly. He came back with the single gene. He knew it right away. He is real aware of it. You know he goes "I don't have to worry about it," and I said "There are some cases you can load a little more iron than somebody else, but don't worry. You will have regular health exams and we will check your levels and go from there." He doesn't feel labeled in any way.
>
> ———
>
> Parents do need to be knowledgeable and make educated decisions for their kids, based on their family history. There are circumstances where certainly it's very important to test, especially if there is disease. If your kids are ill, especially with a treatable disease, then you certainly need to know that knowledge. But then in this case, we weren't going to make any changes based on the information and there were potential downsides. We decided not to test them because of their ages—nine and ten—and the low likelihood of any change in their life based on the findings.

With some exceptions, then, childhood is not a time for susceptibility-gene testing. The exceptions arise when there are obvious health benefits to be gained.

Even when testing is rejected for the time being, parents often face the nagging question of when to tell children about the possibility of a health risk in their future. Informing your relatives that they might have inherited a gene that increases susceptibility to a disorder is seen as a family obligation, as discussed in chapter 4. When and how to tell your own children is also fraught with many uncertainties about how to broach the subject and how to deal with the aftermath.

Some children didn't need to be told because they already knew. Exposure to events unfolding in their families had made them aware of genetic issues.

> My oldest child is eleven now, and so he was very aware of everything when I was being tested for colon-cancer mutations, and I have just kept him very aware of everything and he has been a part of it. He's a witness to the purge every year and actually I think he would go right in and watch the colonoscopy, if the doctor would let him, because he just would love to see his mom's guts. . . . Without shoving it down their throats, I think that growing up with it out in the open like this, it will just seem like a natural thing.

Others learned—or will learn—only when their parents tell them. There are different answers as to when it should be. The time preferred by the parents for this conversation has run the gamut from preadolescence to mid-twenties.

> Before they hit puberty. If I wait until they are teenagers when they are developing themselves then it would perhaps be a scarier experience for them and they will start internalizing that. Whereas if I do it while they are very young, they will have time to process it and by the time they are teenagers perhaps it will be easier.

> ———

> Probably close to adolescence. I don't think children below that age really are capable of thinking about the ramifications of knowing that and what it really means, so I don't think it would be

useful for them to have that information. It could potentially be something they might misinterpret or think there is something wrong with them or "I am different." . . . So probably when they got to the age where they are making a lot of decisions for themselves or beginning to do that, then I would give them that information.

———

Their teen years at the earliest. But if they ask me before then, kind of like talking to kids about sex, I will tell them whatever I can and explain whatever I can before that, but not before their teen years. My fifteen-year-old understands that this information is something that has the potential to keep me safe so that I will have appropriate medical care, and I have been very careful to talk to her about it. I don't want her keeping things inside that I don't know about and if I felt like she needed professional counseling we would certainly get it for her. But I just feel like if we keep talking about it and it's all out in the open I will know what is going on with her. She told me she is glad that she knows and she said it's a good thing, only she didn't want me to tell her friends about it.

———

Not until their twenties. My daughter is in graduate school right now. And she has other things to think about, like trying to get through school and get a job. I don't want her to worry. I would never say anything unless she came to me and said I have to know. My generation is the first generation of people being tested. Most of us are being tested because we have lost somebody to breast cancer. We have either had somebody have breast cancer and live or die and that is why we are being tested. But now it's available to our children too and you know my children have not watched me suffer or die from breast cancer and so they have a very, very different approach to this than I did. And I am really stuck at a crossroads of do I make my issue their issue or do I let them come to it on their own?

Not only must the time be selected to be right for the child but you should also think through what information you will give and how you will give it. It is better to have a plan of action—no matter how tentative—than to leave matters completely to chance. On one occasion, when the awareness arrived unexpectedly, the results were less than ideal:

> I was arguing with my husband. He didn't want me to have testing, saying I was "playing God." While we were arguing, my twelve-year-old daughter overheard and we had to explain it to her. She faltered. She was frightened, and even had to come home from school one day.

Despite divergent opinions about when to tell children, genetic professionals and consumers all agree on one point. There is no one absolutely right time to tell children. It will always be a difficult call.

Decision Question 3: Is This the Right Time in My Life to Be Taking This Test?

To answer this question you must look deeply into your own life. With its many facets and potential for complications, susceptibility-gene testing should probably be embarked upon when one's own life is relatively peaceful. Keep in mind that, even if you feel certain that the time is absolutely right, a temporary or indefinite postponement may be necessary if another family member must be tested first to help find out if there is a family mutation.

There may be reasons to delay, particularly, as we have discussed here, if the testing involves members of the family who have not yet reached adulthood. Unless there are health benefits to be gained from testing children—and hemochromatosis-susceptibility testing might be one such example—testing should not be considered until they are old enough and mature enough to make their own decisions.

With susceptibility-gene testing there is usually no need to rush. The major exception —and one that does introduce some real time pressure—would be when genetic-test results could allow a person already diagnosed with a disorder to decide which of the available medical interventions would be best to take. For example, a woman with breast cancer might opt for a double mastectomy (the surgical removal of both breasts) if she learns that she has a mutant BRCA1 or BRCA2 susceptibility gene, since the presence of that mutation makes a recurrence more likely. Or a man with colon cancer may opt for a full colectomy (surgical removal of the colon) if an HNPCC mutation is found. Often such decisions need to be made promptly so that the surgery can take place with a minimum of delay.

But if you are not faced with an immediate medical decision, forget all those TV medical dramas. It is a good idea to take your time and think carefully about your answer to this question.

CHAPTER SIX

Will the Advantages Gained from Having the Genetic Information Outweigh the Disadvantages?

A Tale of Two Tests

I have had breast cancer, and from my own research I knew there was a genetic test, that there were genes that could be identified for the breast cancer. I had decided I was going to do breast cancer genetic testing because I have a daughter and a granddaughter and I thought that it was of importance to them to see if I did have that identifiable gene. And a lot of people asked me, what are you going to do if it turns out positive? Are you going to have an oophorectomy [ovary removal] or are you going to go ahead and have a bilateral mastectomy [removal of both breasts]? And I said I will get to that, but the most important thing was the hereditary component, and I had had a sister, too, who had breast cancer, and she had two daughters. And so I did it. The test result was actually negative. I did not have bad copies of the BRCA1 or 2 genes. . . . Then my father was diagnosed with Alzheimer's. I guess it became really severe when he said to my mother one day he didn't know who she was. I also knew there was a gene that one might carry for Alzheimer's. The difference here, the reason I didn't pursue genetic testing for Alzheimer's, was because if I had it identified, there really isn't any cure for it. At this stage in my life, I didn't want to know that at some point I was going to encounter it. There really isn't any treatment. There is not a cure for it. So, why make your life more depressing?

—Sonja M., age fifty-nine

In the previous chapters we dealt with three key questions in the decision process. We looked at whether the family history has any telltale signs indicating that you may be at a higher risk for developing a particular health problem, at the kind of information the genetic tests for susceptibility can and cannot provide, and at the timing of the testing. As you think through your decision about susceptibility-gene testing, there is one more crucial question. To answer this question you have to look toward the future to evaluate—as best you can without the aid of a crystal ball—what you will gain from having genetic information. That is, what advantages, benefits, or valuable new options will the testing provide? And at the same time you should estimate—again, doing the best you can—what you might lose, and what kinds of disadvantages, problems, or complications might ensue from having this information. Figuring out the likely impact that genetic information will have on your life is like using an imaginary balance scale, similar to the one the figure of Lady Justice holds in legal settings. On this imaginary scale, the potential benefits of genetic testing are gathered on one pan and the potential disadvantages or harms are collected on the other. When all the items are placed on their respective pans, you then need to see which way the scale tips to help determine whether—for you—the advantages outweigh the disadvantages. It is not just a matter of the number of items that are on each pan, but rather their importance and the extent of the impact they will have on your life.

In this chapter, we will be drawing from the experiences of people who have already considered susceptibility-gene testing for the four disorders that are serving as our examples. (At the risk of being repetitive, we are focusing on hereditary hemochromatosis, breast/ovarian cancer, hereditary nonpolyposis colon cancer or HNPCC, and Alzheimer's disease.) We will also be drawing from what professional geneticists have observed as they have worked with their clients to help them come to testing decisions. Keep in mind that this rich fund of experience can be applied to other genetic-susceptibility tests as they arrive in the clinical setting. The elements that can hang in the balance are organized here in three realms: the personal, the familial, and the societal. Yes, it is necessary that you consider all three realms as you grapple with this question.

Advantages and Disadvantages in the Realm of the Personal

The Advantages

Genetic testing for susceptibility can provide a number of personal benefits. The genetic knowledge gained can help to define one's risk more accurately and may open up a number of different medical options, especially for those found to have a genetic variation that makes them more susceptible to a disorder. These medical options span the spectrum from increased surveillance in order to identify illnesses early, to proactive steps—dietary, chemical, and surgical—that can be taken to reduce that risk, in some cases substantially. Each person must decide, preferably in concert with trusted medical advisers, which actions to take, which to postpone, and which to forgo. There is no single right choice, no "one size fits all" solution. Beyond its usefulness in guiding medical decisions, this type of genetic testing can also offer another advantage: it can provide information that can assist people in the planning of their lives. Let's look more closely at these potential personal benefits.

Risk Assessment and Medical Surveillance. For those who have not been diagnosed with a disorder, a major benefit comes if the susceptibility test reveals one's real risk more accurately. If you have not yet had any disease symptoms but the test reveals that you have inherited a mutant gene that predisposes you to future illness, your higher risk is confirmed. For some disorders, knowledge of the higher risk can lead, in the jargon of the medical profession, to increased surveillance or monitoring. This means more frequent and thorough checkups geared toward detecting the illness in its earliest and most treatable stages. Hereditary hemochromatosis is an example of just such a situation:

> It was because my mom was diagnosed with hemochromatosis and my great grandfather died of—I think it was organ failures—and it seemed like it ran in the family, that I wanted to head it off. My doctor said you can live a long life if you have it diagnosed and

treated early. It's easily maintained if you catch it early. It had not affected any of my internal organs yet, which was a blessing. And so I had a series of phlebotomies [blood removal], one pint a week for nine months and that got all of that excess iron out of my system. Yes, it was really a long nine months, but I was glad to do it because when you hear you have got something serious, it's wonderful to know you can do something about it. Now I am on maintenance so that every three months I get my blood tested and the doctor and I have agreed that if I need a phlebotomy I will get one.

For those who are found to have a predisposing gene for breast/ovarian cancer and colon cancer but have not yet developed the disorder, there are a number of steps that can be taken to help catch the disorder early, when treatments are most effective. These include regular screening (for example, mammographies for breast cancer and colonoscopies for colon cancer), and using these and other diagnostic tools at a younger age than is recommended for women and men who are at the general population risk for these disorders.

Unfortunately, ovarian cancer has no symptoms and the body changes that occur with that cancer are frequently associated with irritable bowel syndrome, flu, or stomach bugs. If a young woman is more aware of ovarian cancer and the ties to herself, she can be more proactive on diagnosis with CT scans [a special form of X-ray imaging]—hopefully catching ovarian cancer in the very early stages. Being educated helps lessen the unknown. Having the chance to make choices gives hope.

———

I knew that if I had a positive result so that I was predisposed to breast cancer, there would be something I could do down the line and right now at least be hypervigilant about monitoring myself.

———

I researched what the recommendations were if you were HNPCC positive. In HNPCC, I think the recommendation is colonoscopies every year or every other year. So, I put my unhappiness with the colon-emptying preparation part aside and that is the route I chose. But I think probably what I am also going to do is CA125 [a blood test for a protein associated with ovarian cancer cells] and CT scans. My goal is to catch it by alternating the tests every six months to try and cover what we can.

In some cases, people felt that the genetic test result, if positive, could help convince insurance companies to pay the costs of the early and more frequent screening—the enhanced medical surveillance—that they wished to have.

Mainly my reason in favor of having the test was to have justifica-tion to get early screening covered by my insurance company.

———

My doctor's recommendation was that the genetic testing be done so that that would then give him the leverage he needed with the health insurance company for the surveillance testing that he would be recommending.

One the other hand, if the test shows that you are a "true nega-tive," that you have not inherited the flawed gene that has been found in your family, it would mean that you are no longer con-sidered to be at high risk. (Remember that "true negative" status can only be obtained when you know the specific mutation that is associated with your family.) You could still develop the health problem, of course, and so it would be appropriate to include reg-ular visits to your doctor and standard screening in your health-management repertoire. However, you would be freed from the need for early and more rigorous scrutiny. Many genetic profes-sionals have found that even with a negative test result, some peo-ple find it hard to shake loose of their former high-risk status and continue to worry that they may still be predisposed to the illness that has been so prevalent for so long in their families.

Reducing the Risk of Illness. Beyond having more intensive sur-veillance that could catch disorders in their earliest stages, there may be additional steps that can be taken to ward off the onset of illness entirely or significantly reduce the chance that it would develop later on in life. They are being shared here to show the range of interventions that have been used and not as an endorsement of any particular approach.

For example, changes in diet are regarded as useful in the prevention of hemochromatosis.

> My number one reason to be tested genetically would be to alter the course of my future, to dodge the bullet, to not come down with hemochromatosis. You could have the genetic disposition, but you could thwart it by diet and donating blood.

Various changes in diet and other lifestyle habits have also been reported to be of some benefit in reducing the risk of different types of cancers and, even, of neurological disorders such as Alzheimer's disease.

For colon cancer, the removal of precancerous colon polyps found during regular colonoscopies can provide an effective means of preventing colon cancer. With breast cancer and ovarian cancer, still other steps are available to reduce the possibility of developing these disorders. Such steps involve the use of drugs (chemo-prevention) such as tamoxifen, which may act to stymie the development of a disease process. Of course, the use of any drug does carry with it the possibility of unpleasant side effects.

Finally, and most dramatically, there is the use of surgery. Surgery can be done to remove an organ that is at risk, before any signs of the disease have appeared. (This is known as risk-reduction surgery or prophylactic surgery.) The preemptive removal of ovaries greatly reduces the risk of ovarian cancer. It also reduces the risk of breast cancer by 50 to 75 percent. The removal of breasts (known as mastectomy) or of ovaries (oophorectomy) or of the colon (colectomy) reduces significantly the risk of cancer from these now-absent organs. But the risk does not away completely. Despite the best efforts of even the most diligent surgeon, some traces of the organ may inevitably be left behind. It should be emphasized that these more aggressive interventions are not suited to everyone. As the experiences of people who have undergone these types of surgery indicate, such decisions are not easy. Each surgical risk-reduction mode has its problems as well as its advantages, and it can be a difficult decision to sort through which, if any, is right for you.

Sue Friedman, the founder of the nonprofit support, education, and advocacy group called FORCE (Facing Our Risk of Cancer Empowered), has often seen the struggle that occurs as people seek to navigate their way through the surgical-prevention options: "I would say the number one issue among the community of women who have been diagnosed with BRCA mutations or other high risk factors is agonizing over whether or not to undergo prophylactic surgery. And these are agonizing decisions. I can't describe enough how poignant and difficult it is to sacrifice a healthy part of your body in order to try and stay healthy and the concerns that go along with that." These decisions take time. But even without time pressure, the decision about how best to lower one's risk can seem overwhelming. The strain is apparent in their words:

> When you think about the test you need to think about what you are going to do afterwards. You are choosing between two evils all the time. It's not like there is one choice that is better than the other. You are really choosing between two evils and that is incredibly hard.

> ———

> I would say, okay, knowledge is power, and I started talking to a lot of people and to as many doctors as I could to get the information, but ultimately I found out it was my own decision. No matter how much information I got, it was still my own personal decision to do it, to have the surgery, or not to do it. You know, when do you stop taking out healthy organs? . . . I said if I did this and then this would happen and I couldn't come to a decision. And then the other side of me would say you have friends going through chemotherapy and you know what they are dealing with, why is the decision so hard?

I could not understand why it was such a difficult decision for me. If I choose not to have the surgery and I got cancer, how am I going to live with myself making that decision? So what I decided at the time was not to make a decision now and to wait ten years until I'm fifty. . . . I would say all this took me almost a full year. . . . And you know it's interesting with me. I felt a lot of anger, and the anger was that I had to make a decision. That is what I felt angry about, that I was faced with a decision. So maybe again, had I known that coming in I could have made peace with that, but I couldn't understand why I was so angry with the whole thing because people always told me that knowledge is power. Now you know and now you can do something about it. I said, "Well I don't feel right" and that was the reason because now I am forced to make a decision to have it or not, and how do I know it's the right decision?

Some women whose genetic test reveals the presence of BRCA1 or BRCA2 mutations do opt for surgical removal of their breasts. This decision, already difficult enough, is frequently complicated by the further need to think through whether to have breast reconstruction and, if they do, which of several reconstruction options would be best.

There was this big cry that women were being mutilated. In my mind I was screaming at those who were saying this. "No, no, don't you understand? If one cell can kill you, they can all kill you." And I don't know why they would prefer to get radiation and chemo. They may have started with a nice set of breasts. I didn't, so that kind of made my decision easier because I didn't have pretty breasts. That is not where my self-esteem was. I could afford it because they weren't pretty and they were lumpy and painful. So for me making a decision about a prophylactic mastectomy was like a no-brainer. I think the women who really wanted reconstructed breasts must have had nice ones to start with and that is a different position to be in. . . . And when I finally had my mastectomy, my surgeon, who had resisted me, came over with my pathology report. I didn't have

breast cancer, but the cell changes they found gave him concern. . . . So at this point I am on surveillance for the ovaries.

Other women have made a different decision. They have opted
for risk reduction for either ovarian cancer or breast cancer by
removal of their ovaries. Here the decision can be complicated by
the additional question of whether or not to remove the uterus
along with the ovaries and whether or not to use hormone
replacement therapy after the surgery.

I decided to do something to reduce my risk of both breast and
ovarian cancer. I knew what my mother had gone through with
ovarian cancer. I saw her suffer, and I didn't want to do that. I knew
there was something I could do that would greatly, not totally, but
greatly reduce my risk, and to me it was a no-brainer. I had the
genetic mutation. I could do this, I was done having children. I
wanted to see them grow up. I was in my mid-forties and I didn't
need my ovaries anymore so it wasn't really a hard decision to have
the oophorectomy. I think the hardest decision was whether I was
going to have a hysterectomy with the oophorectomy or just the
oophorectomy. Well, I talked with a couple of different surgeons. I
talked to my gynecologist, and I talked to other women, and I did
ultimately decide just to have my ovaries out. It was a little overkill I
felt to have my uterus taken out as well. I did start hormone
replacement shortly after the surgery and that was what my surgeon recommended. And I took it for about three years and then I
stopped about a year and a half ago. I have been fine. My bone loss
has been fairly significant, but I started on Fosamax so that was
really the only thing that I noticed. I do monthly breast checks. I do
quarterly clinical exams with different doctors for that, whoever I
happen to be seeing at that moment will do it. . . . So I think what I
might stick with is just doing what I am doing and more mammo-
grams. I feel that what I am doing is enough right now and at least
there are a lot of good screening methods for breast cancer, which
there aren't for ovarian. . . . I feel like I am doing enough right now.

Some women in their quest to reduce their risk as much as possible have opted for surgery to remove their breasts and their ovaries as well.

> I had the genetic test so I could be better informed and better able to manage my own health. And, of course, I had started to think about the "what ifs" before I got the test result, but I didn't put anything into action. Then when I tested positive, the next questions were: Okay, now that you know, what do you do with this type of information? What are the options? Okay God, now what do I do next? And the genetic counselor was able to talk to me in general about different things that people do, you know, the pros and cons of preventative mastectomy and oophorectomy. . . . And I struggled with it. It was a very difficult few weeks. I would come to a conclusion and go no, there has to be another conclusion I can draw from this. But everything led me to the same conclusion, which was the only way to really significantly reduce my risk to where I thought it was acceptable was preventative surgery. I got there, but it was a difficult realization to come to, really emotional and really hard. . . . I decided actually to do everything. I came to the conclusion first on the breast thing, and continued my research and decided the ovaries had to go too. After I made the decision, I set up the appointment with the doctors and scheduled my breast surgery soon after. And then I followed it a few months later with an oophorectomy and actually I ended up getting a hysterectomy too because of complications. Looking back, I have no regrets.

Surgery is a major intervention and there have been some difficulties associated with this type of risk reduction. Removal of the breasts raises issues of body image. Reconstructive surgery, if it is selected, requires that surgical approaches be compared. In some cases, the results from reconstruction are poor, and the surgery may have to be repeated. One woman reported that her reconstruction had to be done three times before she got breasts and nipples that looked natural and did not hurt. And, then too, there is the loss of sensation:

> You know I did have a lot of sexual pleasure from my nipples, and I miss that tremendously, just tremendously. And nobody ever talked about it. I remember before my surgery we were discussing the way the surgery would be, and to me every cell has to be removed and so you should never leave a nipple, never. And my doctor said if you left the nipple you wouldn't have any sensation. That was a huge loss for me, an absolutely huge loss. And, you know, to this day I still really miss that. And nobody talks about it; nobody offers you any counseling about it. It's just this huge void. I mean it's changed our sex life.

Removal of the ovaries—or shutting them down with drugs such as tamoxifen—sets menopause into motion early. There are decisions to be made about whether hormone replacement therapy should be used to relieve the harsher symptoms of menopause since this type of therapy appears to increase breast-cancer risk—an important issue for those who are already at a higher risk.

> The surgery itself was fine. The after-effects, the menopause symptoms, were a drag. I haven't been shy about saying that it's been miserable. You know, right afterwards the night sweats were so miserable. We had to buy a new mattress and I would get no sleep, and I was on an antidepressant for a while for the hot flashes for during the day and just all of that.

For one woman who had preventive surgery to remove both breasts and ovaries, the ovary removal (in her case, coupled with a hysterectomy) was the more difficult procedure.

> It's different when you are put into menopause from surgery versus natural menopause. You have a lot more problems. Nobody could tell me what I was going to be like afterwards until I did the surgery.

You can decide to live without breasts, you don't need your breasts to live, the reconstruction doesn't do anything for you other than cosmetic. But with the hysterectomy, just so many things can change, your whole persona can change. It's something about your essence, you feel so synthetic when it's done surgically, and it's very scary not knowing which one of the effects you are going to wake up with or are going to start happening to you and to what extreme.

Another woman also found the removal of her ovaries a more difficult experience than the surgery to remove her breasts, but for a different reason:

Emotionally the mastectomy is much, much harder. But physically the hysterectomy was way harder than the mastectomy. Oh my gosh, so much harder. Overall, when I had the hysterectomy I got no support from people. I had like fourteen things of flowers when I had the mastectomies and maybe three when I had the hysterectomy.

On occasion, the surgery to remove healthy organs can yield a startling result:

Before the genetic test, I had already made up my mind, based on research I had read, that I would have my ovaries removed. . . . I didn't know what I would do about prophylactic mastectomy, but I knew that I would have my ovaries removed. I didn't need them any more and ovarian cancer is very hard to detect and the surgery is incredibly simple so I had made up my mind. So once I found out I had the gene, my next thought was: All right. So now I have got to find somebody to do this surgery. . . . Fine, he said, but you need to know that in approximately 15 percent of the cases where people go in for this prophylactic surgery, we find cancer. And guess what? The results came back that the first look at my ovaries showed cancer. . . . Yes, it was interesting telling people— because, of course, I had so many to tell—and the message I tried to tell people was how lucky I was because you know this might not have surfaced for another couple of years and, by then, the prognosis would have been very different.

Prophylactic or risk-reduction surgery is also an option when a person is at risk for other types of cancer such as colon cancer. But as Dr. Bard Cosman, a colorectal surgeon and professor of surgery at the University of California, San Diego, explains: "It would not be advisable to perform a prophylactic, or risk-reducing, colectomy [removal of the colon] simply for having a mutant gene, because people with the mutant gene are not certain to develop colorectal cancer, and the operation itself is a substantial one, with the possibility of complications." The men and women who contributed to this book and who were found to have a susceptibility gene for colorectal cancer (or HNPCC) support this view, preferring instead to follow a strict surveillance program, and to have a colectomy only when a cancer or large polyp shows up. The main issue for them has been the key role that the colon plays in the digestive process. Women at higher risk for hereditary colon cancer because of an HNPCC mutation are also at risk for endometrial cancer affecting the lining of the uterus, and they can consider preemptive hysterectomy in lieu of regular checkups.

> I have a colonoscopy every year. I have EGD [visualization of the esophagus, the stomach, and the first section of the small intestine] and an upper GI [gastro-intestinal tract] X-ray every couple of years. I have started going for gynecological testing including like ultrasound, endometrial biopsy, CA125 testing, and I also go for urinalysis and a few other things that affect my kidneys and my ureter because those are two sites where cancer also arose in my pedigree. You know if I were to be diagnosed with a primary colon cancer, I think I would go ahead and have a more aggressive surgery. I would have a total colectomy. But until I am diagnosed with a colon cancer I am going to hang on to my colon.

There is something about your colon. There is just this sort of thing that would give me pause probably because I don't know enough

about it and because it's so much a part of your daily life and functioning. You know I would have to know a lot more. . . . I want to
live, though, so I would listen if somebody told me they thought
that was something I needed to do. I would listen. I don't know
that I would do it.

———————

Ah, that's a big one. That is kind of a thorn in my side from year to
year because my gastroenterologist doesn't pressure me, but he
brings it up every single time, and I like him enough and he likes
me enough that we have an understanding at this point, but he is
very pro-prophylactic surgery. I wouldn't say that I am anti-
prophylactic surgery except for me at this point in my life, I just
really don't feel like it's an option for me. . . . For me it's like this
choice of living in fear. So do I go ahead and have it because I'm
afraid of getting it? It plays into a whole lot of other things for me,
like, you know, spiritual things and how I feel about my body and
sort of living by an "if it ain't broke, don't fix it" kind of thing.

Selecting Treatments. Individuals who have already been diagnosed to have one of the disorders at issue here may also make use
of genetic-testing results to formulate a program of action and
response. For hereditary hemochromatosis, knowledge of the presence of predisposing genes allows those individuals experiencing
symptoms to limit any further damage from that illness generally
through alterations in their diet (to be extremely strict about
reducing iron intake) and phlebotomy or blood removal (to reduce
iron levels already in the body).

I was having a lot of medical problems, arthritis type of problems
with joints and chronic fatigue and all of these other things. I was
just very fatigued all the time, and they just kept blaming it on
stress and working too many hours and just too much stuff going
on with me. Every time they would do some type of testing, but
everything was coming back normal. . . . My iron levels were
higher, but they weren't an alarming signal at the time, so we were

actually having trouble figuring out what was going on. There is really no excuse for somebody my age to feel like an eighty-year-old. Then my brother was diagnosed with hemochromatosis so I was actually anxious to find out if this could be related. I was tested and found to be a compound heterozygote with one copy each of the C282Y and the H63D mutant genes. Now I always have my regular yearly appointments and what not and get my iron checked as a routine part of my regular blood workup, and I just kind of keep track of my ferritin levels and everything else. I was told to keep an eye on my iron, and if it ever gets to a certain level then I need to come in and start treatments like the blood letting. I noticed that when I start getting achy and fatigued and really just start coming down, when I go give blood I tend to feel better.

For people already found to have breast cancer, ovarian cancer, or colon cancer, knowledge of their genetic status can help them make decisions about the best course of treatment to follow. Unlike the situation in which the genetic testing precedes a cancer diagnosis, once such a diagnosis has already been made, treatment decisions frequently need to be made promptly and rapid action may be needed. For many of the people interviewed for this study, their genetic testing came too late, well after the treatment decisions had been made. Several of them felt that they might have chosen differently and gone ahead with more extensive operations had they known about the genetic component of their illness. Freedom from constant worry about recurrence was a familiar theme among the women who had opted for breast and ovary removal following genetic testing.

The surgical oncologist was going to go back in and just take a little bit bigger margin and we would follow up with chemo and then the radiation. I was going to keep my breast. . . . I'm an Ashkenazi Jew, with a family history, and now I have breast cancer. I'm a perfect candidate to be tested. After learning I was positive, I decided to take off both breasts and then, within a short period of time, I took out my ovaries and my uterus also. Everything. . . . You know I have had other people since then talk to me about their particular situation and their torture. I have a girlfriend that comes to mind. Her surgery was two years ago. It was a lumpectomy, and she is being tortured right now. She doesn't feel comfortable. She doesn't sleep well at night, and she now wishes that she had been genetically tested. I think that is one of the things she is wrestling with, and I was telling her, you know there are ramifications health-insurance-wise, but she should consider it. She doesn't sleep well at night because she did the chemo and radiation, and she is not so certain that it isn't spreading. It's a terrible worry, you know. But I sleep peacefully at night. I don't think about it.

—————

Before I always thought about it every day, before I had this genetic testing, every day. I thought about it when I got up in the morning. You know, I had breast cancer, tick tock tick tock, is this the day that I am going to have it again? Every day. And every time I found a little cyst or every time I found a little bump I was on the phone, you know, worrying about it. Now not so much because I have had the surgery, and now I really only worry about it when it's something unusual like my back pain, you know. I don't worry as much because I know it's being taken care of.

Once colorectal cancer develops in a person with the susceptibility gene, then a total abdominal colectomy can be done with the nondiseased portion of the colon being removed along with the diseased portion, under the assumption that it is likely to become diseased in the future. What makes this more extensive surgery a very reasonable option is that the patient is already assuming the risks of a colectomy, and all colectomies have the same operative risk, no matter how much you take out.

I have been having colonoscopies for the last decade because I had a sister who was diagnosed at the age of twenty-six with colon cancer. Last spring when I woke up from my colonoscopy thinking everything was routine, the news was that there was a problem, and that they had taken a biopsy and I would be needing surgery one way or the other regardless. The biopsy came back that it was cancer. It was in the ascending colon, and I did not have my genetic testing done until after I had surgery. They removed the ascending, the transverse, and I think part of the descending colon . . . thinking that that would be prudent. There would be less opportunity for reoccurrence or new cancer because there was less colon. After I had my genetic testing done, and it come back positive, the oncologist said to me that the only thing he would have done differently is that he would have advised me to have my entire colon removed. And I think that would have been a tough call for me. That seemed a bit over the top although it bothers me there is a bit of remaining colon. I feel like maybe it's a ticking time bomb waiting for a new cancer to occur. . . . My impression was that the surgeon would have also recommended removing the ovaries and uterus et cetera at that point when I was having my colon resectioned because of the risk.

Not everyone already diagnosed with breast cancer, ovarian cancer, or colon cancer and found to have a susceptibility gene with a mutation will opt for such extensive treatment. The test has even proven useful in deciding on treatment when a negative result was obtained, as it was for this woman:

I wanted to know if I was at risk for ovarian cancer or not. . . . When I got the negative result, I had mixed feelings, to tell the truth. I thought I would be ecstatic, but in some ways it made my decision-making process about treatment more difficult. . . . Between the time I had the blood drawn and the time I got the results I did some research on my recurrence risk even if I was negative, and I did use the information that I was negative to decide not to have my ovaries out.

The genetic test can be useful for developing an appropriate monitoring plan and for providing the motivation for sticking to it.

Knowledge for Its Own Sake or for Planning Purposes. Another benefit often given in favor of genetic susceptibility testing is that just having information about one's genetic makeup is of value. There are people, sometimes called "information seekers," for whom knowledge itself is important. Having it provides them with a sense of control, regardless of the content. That knowledge might also enable people to plan their lives better. Planning, for instance, can involve decisions about whether to have children or when to have them. For some people, learning of the presence of a susceptibility gene has led to decisions to have children right away so that risk-reduction interventions could be carried out as early as possible, well before any disease process could get under way.

> The very first decision when my test was positive for a BRCA1 mutation was to have children as soon as possible . . . . We were already married, and my husband and I just decided that was enough, you know, inspiration. We just went ahead and started our family. And so I got pregnant right away. When I finished nursing my second little boy, I had my ovaries removed as soon as I could, basically. We were done with our family, done having children.

For others, it has led to decisions not to have children or to adopt children so as not to pass the family mutation on to the next generation.

There is one planning option that did not arise in this study but has been reported in the literature. Some couples are taking the technology of genetic testing a step farther. They have begun to use preimplantation genetic diagnosis, a procedure that allows them to select from among several of their embryos, produced through in vitro fertilization. They can choose the ones that have not inherited the faulty susceptibility gene, and then use only those embryos to achieve a pregnancy. Needless to say, any manipulation of the human embryo raises some thorny ethical concerns. These include concerns arising out of social debates regarding the moral status of the embryo and concerns surrounding the acceptability of selecting against genetic susceptibility to a disorder that may never develop, or that will not develop until decades down the road when medical science is likely to have improved ways of dealing with it.

For some people dealing with Alzheimer's disease in their families, the opportunity to plan seemed a valuable benefit of susceptibility testing.

> I talked with my doctor about getting a genetic test, and he wasn't keen on it. His comment was, "Well, what would you do?" And I said, "Plan." I figured I could plan. I could make sure I got long-term disability insurance. It would prompt me to make plans to do a lot of things through my sixties and seventies if I am in good health. It would make me kind of decide to hunker down and save and not plan on working as long as I had thought I would work.

> ———

> Well, I would probably get much more serious about things that are currently known to prevent Alzheimer's. Although I think I am fairly active mentally, emotionally, and intellectually, I could do more. I could be put on some mailing lists for new information. Right now I am not making it part of my lifestyle to track dementia or Alzheimer's. It's not part of my monthly routine to make sure I am up-to-date on all the things to prevent or all the studies. It's just not on my radar screen as a lifestyle issue. But it would be if I were at risk. I would become much more proactive. I would make sure that I am aware of diagnostic techniques, aware of preventive measures, aware of things I could change and had control over that would give me better odds for stalling or not getting dementia. So, I would be able to address my possibilities directly or more directly. Right now, because I don't know and I have a lot to do in my life, I don't need to be spending my life following up on something that isn't necessary for me to follow up on. . . . But if there was a test and it said you are at risk, that would change my approach instantly. . . . I think it's important for people like me who want to know, to have the right to know. It's not anyone else's decision to make about my right to know my risk factors . . . to make that decision for me. It's my body and my right.

Though many medical professionals offer the view that it shouldn't be necessary for people to take a genetic test in order for them to adopt healthier lifestyles or take time to enjoy life more, the reality is that for many people it would require something like a genetic test result to overcome the inevitable inertia—the tendency to put things off until a later date—that so often characterizes our lives.

The Disadvantages

There are three items that typically appear on the side of not testing. Each of these items parallels the ones that are listed as personal advantages above, but here, as you shall see, they are viewed differently.

The Lack of Medical Options to Deal with Risk. This first item deals with the medical value of the information gained. Will the genetic-test information open the doors for more effective means of treating the illness? Can it help to minimize its damage, or to avoid it altogether? If it does not accomplish any of these things, then, for many, the test results will be of little use. For example, in contrast to the many treatment and risk-reduction strategies available to people with hereditary hemochromatosis and several types of cancer, genetic testing for the Alzheimer's susceptibility gene can help confirm a diagnosis, but it is not particularly useful in deciding on a course of treatment beyond the use of drugs that may, in some cases, slow the progress of this disease. Right now, there is no way to prevent its onset or reverse its course.

> I think the main thing that is holding people back now is the idea there is no cure and at the best you can kind of slow it down maybe a little bit. I am thinking that if a cure or a vaccine presents itself then there will be a flood of requests for the genetic testing.

Susan LaRusse Eckert worked as a genetic counselor at Cornell Medical College and Columbia University on research studies involving genetic testing for Alzheimer's disease. She concurs with this view. In her experience, most people don't really want to know this information primarily because currently they are not going to be able to make changes in their life that reduce their risk. Comfort with Current Surveillance. Even when there are medical interventions to reduce risk, the genetic test may not offer added value. Many people who believe that they are at higher risk are already having regular checkups, in some cases more frequently than the average person. Or they are already taking medication (such as the use of tamoxifen to lower the risk of breast cancer). Or they are already practicing great care with their lifestyle choices. If they are comfortable with their current medical surveillance and do not wish to have prophylactic surgery done and do not plan to change anything they are doing regardless of any genetic test result, then the test has little usefulness to them. After all, they say, if nothing they do is going to change, even if a mutant gene is found, then what additional benefit can be gained from the test?

> Some of my cousins are still in their early twenties and they actually had testing but they just don't want to know the results right now because they said they wouldn't be doing anything different than what they are doing at the moment and they just don't want the burden.
>
> ———
>
> I go every six months to my breast surgeon. I get my annual mammogram. I get a lot of cysts and they can aspirate and drain them or, if they can't, they remove them. So I have had two lumps removed and they have both showed this same precancerous condition. With the oncologist I am on tamoxifen for the next five years, which should decrease my chances of it actually turning into breast cancer by a good 50–60 percent. So that is the route I am going. . . . And when I go in for, you know, an ingrown toenail, I get a breast exam too, and so I probably get a physician-mediated breast exam at least four times a year. . . . I feel I am in good medical hands and that nothing is going to be missed.

Being looked after properly is very important to people who are at higher risk for an illness. For them, it provides the security of thinking that any problem will be caught early, when it is most treatable. In fact, genetic professionals frequently express concerns that receiving a negative genetic-test result might become an excuse for people to become lax about their health-care routines or to slide back into unhealthy habits. And some consumers worry that there is always the possibility that a test result that fails to show a known mutation could be used by health-insurance companies to avoid paying for any enhanced surveillance.

> My daughter does not want genetic testing. Part of the reason, right now she gets the transvaginal ultrasound [a sonogram to view the ovaries] and the CA125 twice a year, and she says if she gets tested and doesn't have the gene, the insurance company will no longer pay for that twice a year. She will go back to a once a year regime. She doesn't want to give that up; she wants the twice-a-year testing.

Emotional Burdens of the Knowledge. The third reason that genetic testing may not be wanted relates to people's attitudes toward medical information. People deal with information—including medical information—in different ways. Some, as we have seen, are information seekers for whom knowledge is power. Information itself is of value and they wish to have as much of it as possible. But for others, medical information may be far less desirable, especially if it brings with it the prospect of endless worry.

> You know, I almost feel better not having genetic testing than knowing, oh my oh my, I have these mutations on these genes. . . . So are you going to sit there waiting for a time bomb to go off? When is it going to happen? Is it going to happen? No, I am not going to live that way.

Family members who have had susceptibility-gene testing themselves sometimes find it hard to understand why their relatives are not equally willing to have that testing too. Often they accuse their relatives of having their heads in the sand or of being in denial. But that kind of criticism may fail to take into account the real psychological costs associated with medical information, particularly genetic information. Some people prefer not to have genetic information so that they may spare themselves the specter of a serious disease looming in their future and so that they may avoid becoming unwilling members of a group sometimes called the "worried well." Nancie Petrucelli, a senior genetic counselor/coordinator at the Karmanos Cancer Institute in Michigan, sums it up this way: "I think it just comes down to your personality and how you cope with the unknown and risk. Some people just don't want to know; they would rather continue going on living as they are, assuming that they are high risk or at low risk. I don't think there is anything wrong with that. It just depends on how people cope with this kind of information. Genetic counselors don't want to do any harm, so ultimately I think it's the clients who must decide what they are equipped to handle."

We have seen in chapter 4 that receiving test results can have an immediate emotional impact. In thinking through the value of genetic information about susceptibility, one must also be sensitive to the longer-term emotional burdens that may come along with any test results.

Advantages and Disadvantages in the Realm of the Family

Advantages

There are benefits of susceptibility-gene testing that go beyond the personal level for the individual considering such testing and have strong implications for the entire family unit.

Informing Children of Their Risk. For many people who are considering susceptibility gene testing, there are clear benefits that can accrue to other family members. Above all, such testing can alert their children to their possible future health risks or reassure them that their risk for a disorder is no higher than it is for the general population. Sonja M., whose interview extract appears at the start of this chapter, was clearly motivated by the desire to inform her children of a potential genetic hazard—susceptibility to breast cancer—that might appear later on in their lives.

If mutant genes that predispose a person to an illness are present in a parent, these genes can be passed on to the children. When the risk is increased by the presence of a single mutant gene—as is generally the case for breast and ovarian cancer, colon cancer, and Alzheimer's disease—then genetic testing of the parent with the disorder (or who is at risk for the disorder based on family history) can establish whether a mutant gene is present. If it is present, then each child would have a 50 percent chance of inheriting that mutant gene at conception. When the disorder is related to the presence of a *pair* of mutant genes—as is the case for hereditary hemochromatosis—then genetic testing of both parents can help establish their genetic makeup and whether or not the children could be at risk. The gene mutations that predispose people to hemochromatosis are common in the general population, so it would not be unusual for two parents to each have such a gene and be able to pass it on without suffering any health consequences themselves. For such couples, there would be a 25 percent chance at each pregnancy that a child would inherit both mutant genes and, thus, an increased risk, later on in life, of hemochromatosis. For many parents, being able to alert their children to such potential health risks is an important benefit of genetic testing.

Once my mom was found to be positive for a breast cancer mutation, which we said we would be surprised if she wasn't, it wasn't a huge choice for me to do it because I have a daughter and I would want her to know if I carried the gene that she has a 50/50 chance of also carrying.

———

Okay, as soon as I felt the lump, I kicked myself and asked myself why didn't I get tested three years ago when I had the mastectomy?

This time, I was tested immediately because I have two daughters and three granddaughters. Now it had urgency because I needed to know if I carried the mutation for my daughters and granddaughters to know. That was absolutely imperative.

———

I would much rather have my children informed so that they would not ignore any kind of warning signals—including the boys. The possibility of breast cancer in males is such a rare thing but I would still like them to be aware of what symptoms might come up, if they come up.

Informing Other Family Members of Their Risk. Within families, as we know, genes are shared not only with children but also with siblings, cousins, and other more distant relatives. Being able to alert these members of the extended family of their risk can also constitute, for some, a real benefit of susceptibility testing.

I made a decision and knew I wanted to have it, and there was very little that anybody else could tell me to persuade me not to have that test because I looked at it as, if I did have this mutation, my sisters needed to know. I was already being watched with a very keen eye for another breast cancer, but my sisters weren't. So I did this mostly so that they would know and be screened more carefully.

———

I really wanted to get genetic testing if it was possible so that the rest of my family could think about their health history in a more productive way. I don't have children, but I have several younger cousins who, even though their dad died of colon cancer and we all had helped to take care of him at home, are really kind of oblivious that it could happen to them. Their defense mechanisms were different from mine, and I felt like if I could show them there really was a genetic basis they might be more careful with their own health, and that was important to me. And they have been actually more careful and are interested in getting genetic testing at some point.

Because hereditary hemochromatosis involves both sides of the family—the mother's and the father's—two sets of relatives may be able to benefit from the test results.

> After my test, my sister got tested for hemochromatosis. It was about 50–50 with my husband's family, about half of them wanting to be tested and half of them not. . . . I would say the people who did, did it more for their children than for themselves.

Some parents were also motivated to test in order to spare their children the stress and strain of having to care for them later on if they could take steps now to prevent the disease itself.

The Disadvantages

Within the family realm, there are items weighing against genetic testing that also need to be considered.

Uncertainty of the Information Obtained. Even with the best of intentions, there is no certainty that genetic information that is useful to others in the family will be obtained. As we have seen in chapter 4, if there is no known mutation in the family, the failure to find a predisposing mutation may not be fully reassuring since other, as yet undiscovered, genes may be involved. Or gene variations may be found, but their meaning with regard to future health may not yet be known. It may be hard to justify going to all the trouble—and expense—of genetic testing if an informative result is not guaranteed.

Uncertainty of Family Reaction. There is no guarantee, even if a specific mutation is found, that others in the family—the children, the siblings, and the more distant relatives who may be at risk—will be grateful for that information. Nor is it always the case that they will act on it by arranging for better surveillance or by seeking genetic testing to determine if they carry that mutation as well. Reactions of individuals within families can—and do—vary markedly. The person who initiates genetic testing is sometimes regarded as a nuisance, pressuring other family members in ways they had not anticipated and causing profound discomfort.

Depending on the individual personalities and their interactions with one another, those who have been tested may have differing degrees of influence on how the information gained through genetic testing is actually used by their relatives.

> They are afraid of what they might hear, you know, and of course that is silly, but I think it's a reality. So I started nagging my cousins on that side of the family, and one young man, the son of one of my first cousins, had been having bad health for years and nobody could figure out what was wrong with him. So when I suggested that he get tested for this, he finally was tested and, yes, he had hemochromatosis too. He is now doing very well.

> When you talk with family members you see different reactions. It's a very personal decision. After my breast cancer gene test, I called each of my siblings and said: "This is what I have done." I was doing it for their kids too. Only my brother said he would pursue it for his daughter. The others didn't want to deal with it. They seemed to think that the issue would go away if they didn't think about it or do anything about it.

> My cousins all made different decisions about the colon cancer gene testing. My oldest cousin was the one diagnosed with cancer so he didn't have the test because he didn't see the point anymore. He assumed it was positive. The second cousin, he immediately ran out and had a full colon examination, which is kind of missing the point. The point is to see whether or not you carry the gene. The third cousin had the test, and she is negative. And cousin four flat out refused to have the test. The reason she gave is because last year she was diagnosed with diabetes. And she decided she already has her disease and didn't want to know about any more.

Substantially different reactions can arise within families following genetic testing and, instead of the better-health decisions that were the original intention, these responses can be the source of ongoing discomfort and dispute. We have already seen (in chapter 4) that survivor guilt can arise when the genetic test results are different for different family members. And parents can feel guilt for passing on mutant genes to their children. Both survivor guilt and parental guilt can become distressing emotional burdens in families in which they occur.

Advantages and Disadvantages in the Social Realm

The Advantages

Usually we do not have to factor in societal consequences—effects that go beyond the individual and the family—when making our own personal health and medical decisions. But, as we have seen, genetic testing is different. There are aspects of genetic testing that connect with the larger society and need to be considered.

Opportunities to Participate in Research Studies. An item for the benefit side of the scale, then, is the use of this testing to contribute to medical research that will enhance our understanding of the genetic component of the illness. Such work might ultimately lead to the development of new interventions that could stop the illness in its tracks. In these relatively early days of genetic medicine, we are only now learning about the long-term consequences associated with particular genetic variations. We are just on the threshold of inventing ways to neutralize the effects of harmful genetic mutations. A great deal more information is needed, and individuals who have had genetic testing and know their genetic status can be sources of valuable information. For some who are considering testing, being able to help the ongoing scientific effort and advance medical knowledge is a positive aspect.

> One of the reasons for testing would be for medical science purposes because there may be a difference between what we know about the H63D gene in hemochromatosis now and how it displays over time— also to educate the medical community of its prevalence.

I don't have children. I decided to go through with genetic testing simply for research purposes because with three sisters and all being married, no one would have put the four of us together for research purposes because we all had different names. So, I brought our relationship to their attention. . . . I just wanted to add to the research data bank and hopefully help somebody else. I mean, sitting with the information was not going to help me, but it might help somebody else.

———

I think I would become more active in Alzheimer's research. I looked around at one point in the mid-1990s at getting into one of the trials that they have for studying people who have immediate family members who have Alzheimer's, but it was a lot of trouble. You had to get all of these tests two or three times a year, go up to NIH [the National Institutes of Health] and be there for a week and all of this business, and it seemed like a big bother. So if I think I knew I was more likely to get it, I would go ahead and do that [to help in] detecting it early and finding better ways to measure what is happening. I think right now the problem early in the onset of the disease is that it's mistaken a lot for depression, for laziness, for different things, and it's really hard for families and physicians for that first year or two when symptoms start showing up.

Participants in research studies usually can expect no direct benefit themselves. But the act of assisting in the advancement of medical science is certainly a noble contribution to the social good, and many people get great satisfaction from doing this.

The Disadvantages

Here we come to something that can be likened to the proverbial elephant in the living room. It is an issue so large that it cannot be ignored or dismissed no matter how hard some may try.

Potential for Genetic Discrimination. This is the issue which was mentioned by nearly every person evaluating the pros and cons of susceptibility-gene testing. There were strong concerns—for some, even deep-seated fears—that the genetic information obtained might find its way into other hands and that once that information is "out," it could be used against them. Insurance companies could use the genetic test results to deny them health insurance or life insurance—or penalize them with vastly higher premiums. Employers, in order to minimize illness-related time loss on the job or to maximize savings in their health care expenditures, could use genetic tests to screen out workers who might be prone to develop expensive illnesses in the future. Government agencies could set genetic criteria that restrict educational or other services. Statements offered by genetic counselors or company representatives to the effect that there have been "no documented cases" of genetic discrimination are not reassuring and, quite often, are simply not believed. People concerned about the disorders that are serving as our model examples had little confidence in the protections provided by the anti-genetic discrimination policies that exist in some states and in the federal-level Health Insurance Portability and Accountability Act (HIPAA). Whether this pervasive skepticism results from knowledge of the historical misuses of genetic information (some of which were mentioned in chapter 1), from direct experience, or from the secondhand reports of the experiences of others is not clear. But what is clear is that fears of the misuse of genetic information are widespread. This was the most frequent reason given for not being tested, by people who stated that otherwise they would have been eager to know the status of their genes. It is also a major worry mentioned by those who already have had genetic testing.

I haven't tried to get health insurance since my hemochromatosis diagnosis so I can't say that I have had any trouble, although I can just about guarantee that it will be a pre-existing condition and that I will have a rate increase, absolutely, which I think is discrimination because I shouldn't be punished for finding out early what I have and treating myself with phlebotomies. And as long as I keep my iron level under control, I am just as healthy as the next person. In fact, I think I am healthier because I do keep up with my blood work. So, if anything, I am probably more on top of my health than the next guy. But the insurance, I am sure, will be higher for me than Joe down the street who wasn't tested.

———————

The whole climate is really an atrocious one, and I think what is happening is that the desire to protect women from revealing this information to their insurance companies keeps us in the closet. It makes it a dirty word, you know. It's like AIDS was way back when. It just seems like it's just a terrible mark against you. It prevents us from reaching out and talking to others, finding other people who may be in the same position and getting support from them. And what I think is the most horrendous part of it is that some women are so afraid to be tested and to have their insurance know about it that they will just go and get a bilateral mastectomy without getting tested. You know it's a flip of the coin. Think of the 50 percent of women who have done that who didn't necessarily have to do it because they might have tested negative.

———————

My doctor [discussing colon-cancer susceptibility testing] also explained that as long as I had my health insurance through my employer and had a group policy, and because of the Health Care Portability Act of 1996, that I didn't need to be concerned about losing my health insurance coverage. However, he did say to me if there ever comes a point in your life where you are self-employed and you find yourself buying health insurance on your own, either they will simply deny you health insurance coverage or the premiums will be very, very expensive.

———————

I talked to my internist about it, and at the time he was telling me that there was testing that could be done but it's one of those things that is two-sided because one thing, you could find out nothing definite—that you were predisposed I guess for getting Alzheimer's—and the other thing is it would be like a preexisting condition for insurance purposes. I guess I just decided not to go any further on it.

You know the costs to industry of health care are enormous, and if there are ways to minimize health-care costs by screening out sick workers, I am sure that there are some companies that would try to do that although it would be highly illegal. I am sure it would still happen. . . . And I am sure in the future, as we have more systematic databases available for health care, that hackers will get into them and data will become more available. I have no doubt about this. And so over the twenty-to-fifty-year time frame that's relevant here, I suspect that our ability to get and keep a job will depend on our, in part, on our health-care reports. So you have to be very careful what gets in there.

People are concerned not only about themselves and their own insurance coverage. That pesky reality about genes—that they are shared in families—leads to worries that genetic tests of parents could also label their children, and eventually lead to discrimination against the children at some point in the future.

I don't want hemochromatosis to get on her medical record when she is seven years old because I am worried, what if she gets turned down for health insurance when she is on her own? Right now she is under our policy; that is not really a concern. . . . I am thinking for the future for when she is out on her own and wants to get insurance. If that has been on her record since she was seven—you know, hemochromatosis, . . . I don't want her to get labeled with that. Am I wrong thinking of that?

—————

My sister is extremely afraid of insurance discrimination, more so not for her, but for her daughter. She has a nineteen-year-old daughter, and she is afraid that it will affect her insurance later in life. So that is why she will not do it. She refuses to have it done.

These fears about genetic discrimination, which arose again and again in the oral histories collected for this study, have led people to take matters into their own hands. They have done so in a number of different ways by

- deciding to pay for the genetic testing themselves, or undergoing testing anonymously using false names and bogus identifying information—all of this done so that the test result cannot be traced back to them;
- arranging, with the permission of their doctors, to keep the genetic test results out of their regular medical records or for a so-called shadow file to be kept separate from their medical records, thereby keeping genetic information away from the prying eyes of insurance companies or employers;
- making all the testing arrangements themselves, independently of the medical community, through the use of testing laboratories (usually found via the Internet) that provide direct-to-consumer testing;
- altering their life's dreams of starting their own businesses or taking early retirement, or otherwise reconfiguring their career goals so that they can always be under the protection of (and, hopefully, hidden within) a group insurance plan.

As creative—or desperate—as these attempts are to insulate oneself and one's loved ones from suffering the harms of genetic discrimination, they can lead to a number of problems. Insurance companies may not be willing to pay for extra surveillance or for the use of risk-reduction surgery without genetic-test evidence that the individual is at a higher risk. Incomplete or inaccurate medical records could lead to misdiagnoses or less-than-optimal treatments, especially in situations in which the official medical records have been transferred to physicians who are not familiar with the patient. Those who arrange all the testing on their own can find themselves at the mercy of direct-to-consumer organizations, some of which may be out for a quick profit and not organized to deliver high-quality services or to provide effective follow-up recommendations. And while giving up on a life's dream because of fears of genetic discrimination may not seem as significant as these other problems, it's always a major blow to the people who feel they have been forced to make such a sacrifice.

A final wrinkle on the insurance issue is this: some people are put off genetic testing by what can only be called the "health-insurance hassle." This hassle consists of the need for seemingly endless contacts with insurance companies to gain approval for genetic testing, for surveillance plans, or for risk-reduction surgery. The endless back-and-forth of requests, rejections, and reconsiderations—not to mention phone calls, letters, and physician pleadings—can be an exasperating experience. For one individual whom I interviewed, the approval for a prophylactic mastectomy came only hours before the scheduled surgery. In such a user-unfriendly environment, people have given up out of frustration or exhaustion.

At present there are a number of state laws and sections of federal laws that offer protections against some forms of genetic discrimination. Despite this, the fear of discrimination continues to be a major barrier to the pursuit of susceptibility-gene testing. A new, more comprehensive piece of federal legislation, the Genetic Information Nondiscrimination Act (GINA), may help allay consumer concerns about health-insurance and employment discrimination. GINA is discussed in chapter 9 (pages 139–141).

Decision Question 4: Will the Advantages Gained from Having the Genetic Information Outweigh the Disadvantages?

As we have seen, this is not an easy question. There are different facets to explore, and they involve not only the potential advantages and disadvantages of susceptibility testing (as we have discussed) as well as their likely magnitude and impact, but they also involve the factoring in of the special features and realities that characterize your own life. You will also notice that each type of susceptibility testing requires its own type of evaluation. What you conclude for one disorder may not be the same for another disorder. Sonja M., whose words appear at the start of this chapter, decided that the balance was in favor of breast-cancer susceptibility-gene testing but decided exactly the reverse for Alzheimer's-susceptibility testing. It is tempting to look for a shortcut and rely on how others have answered the question. However, since no two life stories are alike, it would be a mistake to import someone else's conclusion, plug it into your own situation, and hope for the best. There really is no substitute for figuring it out for yourself.

But there may be ways to get some help as you think through this and the other three key questions. In the next chapter we will find out how to gain assistance in the decision process.

CHAPTER SEVEN

Decisions, Decisions

Opposing Decisions

My father and several of his relatives had died of colon cancer, but he always said there wasn't a genetic link. He blamed it on their diet, that they ate a lot of foods fried in lard. But a cousin was tested and they found a colon-cancer gene. I was just born for the Internet. I love having all of this information available to me, and I searched out information and decided to have genetic testing myself to find out my chances for getting colon cancer. The major reason is I have three children. I couldn't cope with knowing or not knowing if I had this gene and passed it on to them. I wanted to know. I am naturally inquisitive, I guess. The genetic test showed that I do not carry the gene, that I don't have it. I won't develop the disease from the genetic part. The report said you can still get colon cancer, but it won't be the genetic family disease.

—Arnold T., age forty-five

I have become convinced that I probably have a high risk to have colon cancer. My father and his sister and her son all died from it. I may be the next one in line. It has started becoming kind of real to me. But I haven't wanted genetic testing. You really have to think about how it will affect you. I hesitate because I know that if you were to get positive results there are so many decision points. And I worry that I won't be able to do the things they want. Let's say, for example, they wanted me to have a colonoscopy every so often. I don't know if I could even pull that off. Who would order it? Would my insurance be willing to pay for it?

—Barbara T. (Arnold T.'s sister), age forty-eight

One family. Two siblings. And yet Arnold and Barbara came to two different conclusions about having genetic testing for susceptibility to colon cancer. How can this happen? Unlike the other tests available at our doctors' offices, whose use is usually left to the good judgment of our health care providers, your input is crucial to the genetic-testing decision. It is not advisable to simply follow, in lock step, what other family members do, or to succumb to the pressure exerted by others. Decisions about these new genetic susceptibility tests must be made by each person individually. You need to answer for yourself each of the four key questions discussed in the preceding chapters and, based on those answers, come up with the decision that suits you best. The decision requires reflection on the realities of your life, your personal values, your attitudes toward risk, and your commitments, strengths, and fears. There is no magic wand to point us to the perfect path, no oracle from Delphi who can tell us what to do. Nobody else knows your life circumstances better than you do, and nobody else will have to live as closely with the consequences of your decision. The choice—whether to have testing, not to have testing, or to postpone the testing decision to some future time—must be yours.

Decision Basics

For readers who have answered "yes" to each of the four questions posed here, conditions may be reasonable—or as reasonable as they can be—for going ahead with susceptibility testing.

For readers who have answered "no" to one or more of the four decision-guiding questions, the conditions do not appear right for proceeding with susceptibility-gene testing. Conditions can change, of course. If over time, significant changes occur, these could trigger a reevaluation of the original decision. For example, later on you might obtain better information about the family health history. The new information you acquire might significantly increase the likelihood that a hereditary component is involved. Or a relative who has had the disease may later decide to undergo testing to see if a susceptibility-gene mutation is present. Or the complexities of life that were decisively distracting earlier may abate, providing a now favorable time for testing. Or medical options may arise that offer new means, more effective or more acceptable to you, to defend against future illness. As you can see, it is always possible that changed circumstances can cause your assessment to change and convert what had been a "no" into a "yes." As a result, you should be prepared to rethink your original decision periodically to see if changed conditions might alter your answer. Whatever the circumstances, the decision must be yours.

For some people in this study who forged ahead with genetic testing even when one or more of the guiding questions met with a "no" answer, there have been some unsatisfying outcomes:

- Without evidence of a family history of a disorder (a question 1 issue), testing was ultimately viewed as a huge waste of time and money.
- There was severe disappointment when, in the absence of a known family mutation, the genetic test yielded a negative result that left the clients with the same uncertainty they had before undergoing the test (all part of question 2).
- Testing at an inopportune time left a residue of wounded feelings and strained family relationships (what we looked at in question 3).
- And proceeding with genetic testing without considering the anticipated advantages and disadvantages (what we were trying to figure out in question 4) produced lingering regret and family problems.

Unless urgent medical-treatment decisions require that genetic testing be done rapidly, it is important not to rush the decision process. One person recommends a laid-back approach:

You can't go with your heart because your heart doesn't always think straight. Your heart feels, your brain thinks. And when you can't seem to make a decision and are trying hard to make a decision, stop trying. Get the data, figure out how you feel, and stop thinking about it. Let it marinate. . . . Some people get very, very frightened and that overrides their ability to decide. So just letting it sit on the back burner for a while seems to help.

For another individual, it took five years to reach a satisfactory conclusion about what she wished to do. All along the way, she bounced back and forth between yes and no. And what you decide about susceptibility testing for one disorder may be quite different from what you decide about another. Each type of genetic testing should be considered on its own merits using the four questions presented here.

Genetic professionals have all experienced the situation in which a person proceeds with susceptibility-gene testing and then decides not to get the test results. Though the client had left a sample for genetic testing, he or she never came back for the test results. This has also happened in the Alzheimer's disease research studies. Participants who indicated that they were eager to get their genetic results at the start of a study later turned down the chance to learn their genetic status when it was offered to them at the study's end. It's okay to change your mind like that. You can decline the results at the last minute, if you decide to. But once you receive the results, it's too late to decide not to know.

Decision Assistance

Though you have to arrive at your decision independently, this does not mean you need to make it in isolation. Many of the people whose experiences informed this book sought assistance as they made their way toward their own decisions.

A clear and obvious first step when deciding on a genetic test is your own physician. Here the term "physician" is broadened to include the family doctors and the various medical specialists who have cared for you over time and who may have come to know you quite well. For people who are most comfortable with a trusted physician, this can be a valuable place to turn. However, a recurring theme throughout our interviews (and in the professional literature as well) is that many doctors are not yet well informed about genetic testing in general and about the newest genetic tests for susceptibility in particular. As a result, some doctors may not pick up on the possibility of a genetic cause for a disease that appears often in a family, and they may be unfamiliar with the psychological and societal dimensions of genetic testing. Then too, physicians are burdened with many demands on their time. Nowadays the typical office visit with a doctor is usually only a few minutes, far too short to allow much progress to be made on something as complex as a genetic-testing decision. Medical doctors are trained to work in a more directive fashion. In fact, that's what most people expect from their doctors. They want the doctors' best advice, "doctor's orders." It may be difficult for physicians to take a neutral stance while discussing the many different facets of the genetic testing decision. Nonetheless, for many individuals, the interaction with their doctors has been extremely helpful.

> My doctors all said to me, you are doing the right thing if this is what you want to do. It's your decision. But they also sat down and talked to me about what my options would be if we found out that I didn't have the mutation. We had those discussions long before I had the test because I need time to get used to things, so I wanted to know what I would be facing should this test result come back as a mutation.

Others found their physicians to be less helpful. Several consumers received contradictory advice from their doctors.

> My doctors disagree about colon-cancer gene testing. When I mentioned it to my gynecologist, she was very discouraging about it. She thought it was a bad idea in that there wouldn't be much she could do about early detection and she felt that it would not

really accomplish anything. Whereas the gastroenterologist, once I brought it up to him, he actually thinks it's a good idea, and he thinks I should do it . . . . It's just been very confusing to me.

Check with your doctors to make sure they have detailed and up-to-date knowledge of susceptibility tests, and also have the time to help you decide. Often other members of your doctor's staff can step in to be of assistance. For example, nurses, particularly those who specialize in oncology, have had training in genetics, are aware of the intricacies of the testing process, and can make more time available to you during your decision process.

Certainly another obvious source of expertise are the genetic professionals themselves, particularly genetic counselors. Genetic counselors are trained to help people make decisions and to do so in a neutral, nondirective, fashion. This means that they do not recommend for or against testing, but instead serve as information providers and sounding boards to help their clients reach a decision. These professionals typically spend a significant amount of time with each client. Genetic-counseling appointments can run for an hour or longer, and genetic counselors remain in regular contact with their clients throughout the decision process. Obtaining assistance from these professionals assumes that the client has been considering testing within the framework of a genetics unit and is prepared to pay, out of pocket or through insurance, the extra cost associated with this specialized service. Recall that, in this study, only about half of the consumers had any contact with genetic professionals as they made their genetic-test decisions.

A potential source of advice and assistance are psychologists or licensed counselors. It is very likely that psychologists or counselors may themselves not be versed in genetics or familiar with susceptibility testing. Despite this, they are well experienced in helping people make decisions. They can be of particular use in helping you sort through the emotional and family issues that might arise, especially if they know how you have faced crises in the past and how you have coped with challenges. Such insights can be a good help in advancing the decision process.

Whenever you consult with any health-care professional, a number of steps will help you to get the most out of that interaction and ensure that you get the best information possible:

- Be sure that you are fully dressed (not in some flimsy paper garment you may have worn if there was a physical examination) and seated in a real office (not in a treatment room) so that you are comfortable and the conversation is on an equal footing.
- Come prepared with questions. Then ask more questions. And if you don't understand any of the answers, ask again. Too often we are reluctant to do this for fear of looking unintelligent. But a genetic-testing decision is, by its very nature, extremely complicated. Restate in your own words what you have heard ("So you are saying that . . ." or "Let me repeat what you said to be sure that I understand"). You want to avoid any chance of misunderstanding.
- Ask for alternative explanations, especially if numbers, such as probabilities and statistics, are involved.
- Take notes. If you can, use a tape recorder to capture the whole conversation. You may be surprised when you listen to the tape at a later time that there were some key items that you missed. If you can, invite a trusted person to be there with you. What one person misses, the other person will likely get.
- Ask for a written summary of what transpired during the meeting and take home with you any educational materials that were provided. You can study all these materials at your leisure.
- Before you leave, be sure to find out whom you should contact if you have further questions or need more information.

Some consumers have turned to another resource in sorting out their testing decision: family and friends. The results here, understandably, range from extremely helpful to, well, not so helpful. In these oral-history interviews, two major stumbling blocks were noted. First, genetic susceptibility testing is an area with which most people are unfamiliar, so most people have no basis for giving advice to others.

> People who don't have the risk are not as supportive as they want to be. They kind of don't have a clue.

> They can't understand because they've never walked in my shoes, since it's not that common. And I don't think people can help you unless they are in your position or are very familiar with genetic counseling, or if it's somebody who has had the test.

> The people that I know, people from work and that sort of thing, they just have the sort of deer-in-the-headlights thing. Run for the hills. It's not something they want to talk about.

The other stumbling block that can arise comes from the fact that genes are shared in families. Your decision can hit uncomfortably close to home for relatives of a person considering genetic testing. Family members advising a relative may face the possibility that your genetic testing could have implications for them as well. This discomfort may color their advice or cause them to withdraw from conversation.

> My parents do not want to discuss this. They don't want to hear about it. My family does not want to hear about it and they don't want to be hounded about it and talk about it.

A particularly useful aid to your decision making can come from a group of total strangers who don't know you and whom you may never meet in person: members of support groups. Over the last several decades, support groups set up by people dealing with—or concerned about—serious illnesses have become an important feature in the world of health care. Either at face-to-face meetings or via the Internet, support-group members provide one another with information about shared illnesses and offer practical suggestions for dealing with them. Some groups also raise money to support scientific research on their condition. These groups encourage a sense of community among those who are faced with the same health issues—wherever they may be—and they help overcome the isolation that often accompanies serious illnesses. Groups typically have an advisory board of medical experts to help answer technical questions that arise. Support groups come in all sizes. Some have many members and operate a Web site that offers the latest information on the disorder and an opportunity for on-line discussion. Others are quite modest in size, and still others may be a few individuals communicating from time to time on a discussion board.

In their most recent incarnation, support groups have been established as a resource for those who have a predisposition to an illness but who haven't developed it. These support groups are helpful in bringing together people who are dealing with—or have dealt with—the same types of decisions about genetic testing that you are facing. These are people who have, indeed, walked in your shoes and shared your concerns. However they are organized, support-group members can facilitate the decision-making process by listening to your concerns and sharing their own, often hard won, expertise.

One such group, FORCE (Facing Our Risk of Cancer Empowered), was begun in 1998 as a safe haven for those at higher risk for breast and ovarian cancer. According to Sue Friedman, the founder, "These women were kind of in their own little limbo because they had been diagnosed with risk and not cancer, and these women seemed very uncomfortable going to cancer-support sites with all of these people who were going through chemotherapy and radiation." As a means of self-identification, FORCE uses the term "previvor" to describe someone who is at high risk for a disorder that has not yet developed.

The FORCE Web site and the associated telephone help line now get hundreds of thousands of hits per month. This has been useful for many in advancing decision making related to breast cancer and ovarian cancer on everything from genetic testing to risk-reduction strategies. One of the women I spoke with put it this way:

> At FORCE, the women support whatever decision you are making. They just want to support an intelligent well-thought-out process for you to make your decision, and that is its culture. Sometimes you have to go over these things over and over again in your head. When you are frustrated by this or that problem or the insurance, you can burn out the people in your environment really, really fast for the amount of venting you need to do. With FORCE, I can vent and they can validate. So FORCE is great.

Each of the four disorders that we are using as examples have similar types of support groups. It is certain that the number of groups for other disorders will increase along with the development of new susceptibility tests. Ways to find support groups are included in the Resources section at the back of the book.

As helpful as support groups can be, it is important to choose carefully. Whether it's a local group with regularly scheduled meetings or an Internet site that you can log onto whenever you wish, you should find out first if it will suit your needs. Groups intended for people who have already been diagnosed with the disorder may not be as welcoming to people with a genetic predisposition. The Internet can be useful, but it is also awash in incorrect information, outdated material, and biased sources out to persuade you to buy a particular product or use a particular genetic test or testing service. Try to determine how the advice that is being presented has been arrived at. Does it reference recent and reputable research? Does it provide information about a number of different options? Is there an advisory board of people, consumers and professionals, with first-rate credentials? It is well worth your time to investigate and be sure that it's the right place for you.

And What If Your Decision Turns Out to Be Wrong?

There is no guarantee that any decision you make will be completely free of problems or will yield no unpleasant surprises. For example, if you opt for the genetic test, you may discover that your own reaction to the results may be stronger—or last longer—than you expected. Or you may discover that other family members may be less supportive than you thought they would be. It may turn out that the balance of advantages and disadvantages that you worked hard to estimate may play out differently in real life from what you had imagined.

You cannot fault yourself if things don't turn out exactly as you expected. All you can do is make the best decision you can with the information available to you. No one can expect more.

CHAPTER EIGHT

Deciding about Other Types of Genetic Tests

Three Vignettes

Erika, thirty-nine years old, is finally pregnant. It has taken nearly a year of visits to an infertility clinic, and she and her husband, Tim, are ecstatic. At her first prenatal care visit, her obstetrician mentions that Erika is at a higher risk for having a child with Down syndrome. Erika is stunned. "How can that be?" she says. "Everyone in my family is healthy, and in Tim's family too. No one has anything like Down syndrome." Then she wonders how she might find out if her baby has this condition.

Ted's cousin and best friend since childhood has cystic fibrosis. Over the years Ted never thought much about this disease—until now. He plans to propose to his college sweetheart. But some nagging thoughts have begun to surface: Does he carry the mutant gene? Should he be tested? And when should he share this information with the woman he loves?

Dawn and her husband, Brian, have made an appointment with a genetic counselor. Dawn has recently learned that Huntington disease has been diagnosed in her first husband's family and that Alexis, Dawn's daughter from that marriage, is at risk. Brian insists that Alexis be tested to see if she has inherited the gene. He tells the counselor: "If she has the gene, I want to be prepared. I will begin to set money aside now that can be used to help provide necessary care for her whenever the disease makes its appearance."

Genetic-susceptibility tests have been the main focus of our attention thus far. But there are other kinds of genetic tests. Maybe you
are pregnant and your doctor has told you about prenatal genetic
tests that can reveal whether or not your fetus will be born with a
particular genetic disorder. It may be that a close family member
has been diagnosed with something, such as sickle-cell anemia or
cystic fibrosis. You wonder about a genetic test that can tell you
whether, hidden away in your genetic makeup, is the specific
mutant gene that is associated with that diagnosed disorder. Or it
may be that you have a family history of a genetic disorder—one
that appears later in life—and you are wondering about a genetic
test, a presymptomatic test, that can tell you right now whether or
not you will develop that disorder in the future.

It would be natural to ask if the same four questions that we have
emphasized, the key questions entering into decisions about genetic
testing for susceptibility to common health problems, could also be
used to help make decisions about other types of genetic tests. The
answer is yes. The four questions are also useful when other types of
genetic tests are considered. Not surprisingly, given the variety of
genetic tests available and the variety of situations that surround
such tests, new aspects arise that will need to be taken into account
when answering these questions. Conversely, some concerns that
arose with susceptibility-gene testing will loom less large with other
forms of genetic testing. Regardless of the details, the template for
guiding the decision-making process remains the same.

Let's look at how the four questions play out in the context of
other types of genetic tests: prenatal tests, carrier tests, and
presymptomatic tests (or, as they are also called, predictive tests).

Prenatal Genetic Tests

Until recently, very little was known about the fetus until the
moment of birth. In fact, much of the excitement surrounding the
birth of a baby had to do with finding out if the new addition was a
girl or a boy and if the baby was healthy. Nowadays, there are many

techniques that are capable of acting like tiny searchlights to probe this previously hidden world. For example, the use of ultrasound has made it possible to look into the womb and identify features associated with the normal progress of fetal growth and development. Ultrasound scans can also identify the anatomical signs associated with each sex, so that expectant parents can learn, early on in the pregnancy, whether the new baby will be a boy or a girl.

Prenatal genetic tests can go even further and reveal details about specific inherited traits of the fetus. There are procedures—amniocentesis and chorionic villus sampling being the most common—that collect and analyze a small sample of cells produced by the fetus. These cells, each of which contains the complete collection of genes of the fetus, can be analyzed in different ways. It is important to keep in mind that these cell-collecting procedures are not without risk themselves. In a very small percentage of cases, there are complications that can bring about the spontaneous termination of the pregnancy.

In the laboratory, the fetal cells can be treated so that their chromosomes—the rodlike structures containing the genes along their length—are made visible in through-the-microscope photographs. This allows the total chromosome number and the structural integrity of each individual chromosome to be determined. Humans have 46 chromosomes. If there is a different number of chromosomes, it is a strong signal that there may be health problems. For example, Down syndrome results when there is an extra chromosome 21 present. Should there be a chromosome with a structural defect, so that it is either missing genetic material or has extra genetic material, this too can contribute to a variety of health problems. The fetal cells can also be examined for specific mutant genes—genes whose presence is an indication that the baby may be born with a disorder such as cystic fibrosis or Tay-Sachs disease or sickle-cell anemia. Hundreds of genetic tests are available that can identify the specific mutations associated with specific diseases. Most of these tests provide information about diseases that are considered "rare." Many are so rare that most people are unfamiliar with their names. They affect far fewer people than do the susceptibility genes connected with common diseases. Added together, of course, these rare disorders reach into the lives of significant numbers of people. When they do appear they can place heavy burdens on the individuals coping with them, as well as on their families.

As you think about whether to proceed with prenatal genetic testing, with our four questions as the guide, the first thing to establish is whether the fetus might be at a higher-than-average risk for a particular disorder. Since prenatal genetic tests don't test for every possible flaw, you have to know in advance what you're looking for. Do not rely just on the "genetic grapevine"—that informal combination of family lore, hazy recollections, and often outdated medical information—that exists in many families. An accurate and current family medical history (as described in chapter 3)is as important a prerequisite for prenatal testing as it is for susceptibility-gene testing. A trained genetic professional or a genetically savvy physician can use this medical history to spot a possible pattern from what may seem to be unrelated illnesses in different corners of a family. Or something that was left unspoken—the early death of a child, perhaps—may prove helpful in tracking the path of a flawed gene through a family network.

Other factors may also indicate the possibility of increased risk for a chromosome or gene disorder:

- Information from routine ultrasound scans and blood tests done during a pregnant woman's visit to her doctor can reveal anatomical or chemical features that raise concern.
- Age needs to be considered. As a woman ages, errors in the chromosome number of her eggs tend to occur more frequently. This is why Erika, 39, in the first vignette, is at a higher risk for having a child with a condition such as Down syndrome.
- Members of specific ethnic and heritage groups are at higher risk for some types of genetic disorders. Cystic fibrosis, for instance, appears more often in Caucasians. Tay-Sachs disease occurs more frequently in individuals of European (Ashkenazi)

Jewish heritage. African Americans whose ancestors once lived in malarial regions of Africa are at a higher risk for sickle-cell anemia. In fact, every ethnic and heritage group has some disorders—or gene mutations—for which its members are at a higher risk

All of these must be considered as you try to determine if your fetus might be a candidate for prenatal genetic testing.

But heightened risk alone is not the only factor here. There are some inherited conditions that are relatively minor. For example, there is a genetic mutation located on the X chromosome that results in colorblindness. Other than causing a person to make the occasional odd color choice in clothing, or to mismatch a pair of socks, this is not a serious problem. Despite any raised colorblindness risk based on family history, it is generally ignored. For other genetically based illnesses, the symptoms may be so mild—or the available treatments so effective—that people may prefer just to wait and to deal with the problem if and when it arises. If the probability is low that the fetus has inherited a mutant gene (or pair of genes) or an incorrect number of chromosomes, it may not be worth risking the pregnancy from possible complications of the fetal-cell-collecting procedures involved in prenatal testing.

As we saw in chapter 4, the next question that needs to be considered en route to a genetic-testing decision is whether the test will provide useful information. The fetal-chromosome picture (also called the karyotype) can reveal whether there is an error in the number of chromosomes, or if there is another visible chromosomal anomaly. Equally important, the karyotype can indicate that, from a chromosome-number and structural standpoint, everything seems fine. Either way, parents will be receiving useful information. But no test is perfect, and if there are very small changes in chromosome structure, they may not be detected.

When it comes to a disorder brought on by a single mutant gene (as in a dominant disorder such as neurofibromatosis) or by a pair of mutant genes (as in a recessive disorder such as cystic fibrosis), genetic tests can establish just what genes are present. But even with the sophisticated tests that current genetic science now provides, there are some difficulties. For many disorders, flaws in any one of several different genes may be responsible for the very same symptoms. It does no good for a test to examine the status of gene A if it is really gene B that is at fault. Moreover, any one of several different flaws in the same gene can interfere with the gene's function. This means that genetic testing needs to be done first on family members who may have the mutant gene. This will help to identify which specific gene is flawed and which mutation is involved. Then, that mutation can be targeted in the subsequent genetic testing of other family members, including the developing fetus.

When it is established that certain specific mutant genes are present in the family, one or both parents must be tested first before any testing is done on the fetus. Examination of the parental genetic makeup will reveal if particular mutant genes are actually present. (If they aren't there, there's no need to test the fetus.) For dominant disorders, a single mutant gene in either parent raises the fetus's risk of inheriting that gene (and developing the disorder) to 50 percent. For recessive disorders, both parents must be carriers of the mutant gene for the fetus to be at risk. If they are both carriers, then there is a 25 percent chance at each pregnancy that the fetus will inherit both mutant genes (and develop the disorder). There is certainly no point in putting the fetus at risk from testing if the mutant gene is not present in the parents.

If prenatal testing does proceed, the genetic tests used can probe the status of individual genes and tell whether these genes are flawed. If the test shows that only one mutant gene for cystic fibrosis, or Tay-Sachs disease, or sickle-cell disease is present, then the baby will be a genetic carrier for that disease but will not get the disease. However, if the test reveals that two mutant genes are present, then the baby will be born with—or later develop—the symptoms of that disease. Unlike susceptibility-gene tests, where the tests can supply only a probability that an illness may appear someday, prenatal tests are more definite. The presence of chromosomal anomalies or gene mutations in a prenatal test is usually a nearly certain indicator of future health status. Even so, it cannot always be determined just when the disorder will appear or just how severe it will be.

There are a few prenatal tests in which the results may not be definitive. It is not always possible to determine if a particular variation found in the DNA will have an effect, or if a structural alteration found in the genetic material is extensive enough to cause health problems. Sometimes genetic information is obtained from linkage testing, in which a trackable DNA landmark located near the gene of interest is used as a marker to signal its presence. Information gained from a linkage test contains some built-in uncertainty because the connection between the marker and the target gene is sometimes disrupted by the tendency of genes to occasionally cross over to a position on the partner chromosome.

As we have seen in chapter 4, the period of time awaiting genetic-test results can be filled with much anxiety. This anxiety is intensified for prenatal testing since the test results concern the health of one's future child. For many parents-to-be, this is an achingly difficult time. It is important how the testing is conducted. A careful evaluation of your family health and genetic history should be carried out beforehand. If prenatal genetic testing is then done, it is essential that there be one or more careful follow-up sessions in order to digest and fully understand the results. On a practical note, you should also know in advance what the costs will be for these sessions and for the testing, and what part of these costs you must pay for yourself.

The question of timing—as we have discussed in chapter 5—is important here. Compared with most other types of genetic testing, the window of opportunity for prenatal testing is very narrow. The techniques for acquiring a sample of fetal cells can only be performed at specific times. Chorionic villus sampling can only be done between the tenth and twelfth weeks of the pregnancy, when the chorionic villi are present. Amniocentesis is carried out a bit later, typically between fourteen and eighteen weeks of the pregnancy. Mindful of these time restrictions, people considering such testing will need to be prepared to decide more quickly than they might otherwise like. Some people start working on their health histories and arrange for genetic testing to determine their own genetic status well before a pregnancy has begun. They do this so they will have the maximum amount of time to think through their decision about proceeding with prenatal genetic testing.

In addressing the last question in the decision template, it is necessary, as we saw in chapter 6, to figure out whether the advantages of prenatal genetic testing outweigh the disadvantages. Prenatal genetic testing offers some new elements to consider here. For many, the test results will be reassuring: a normal chromosome complement will be found or the gene mutation will be absent. These results, of course, don't guarantee that the fetus will be born healthy, only that the fetus won't have the disorder that the genetic test targeted. Nonetheless, genetic-test results can relieve prospective parents of a great deal of anxiety.

Sadly, for others, their worst fears will be realized if the test results show that genes associated with a particular illness have been passed along to the fetus, or if the chromosomal picture that is obtained is not the standard one. As painful as it is to learn that their as-yet unborn child will have to deal with health problems, either from birth or in the years that follow, once their initial shock has subsided, many prospective parents have found that even such unwelcome test results provide a real benefit: it gives them extra months to begin planning. Parents have made use of this window of time to learn about the kinds of health problems their child will face and to determine what sorts of medical care will be needed. They have been able to line up medical specialists and other health professionals who can work with them to ensure that the correct care begins promptly. It has allowed parents to explore what educational and other services are available in their communities, and to find out what support groups can be of help to them. Overall, the information from a prenatal genetic test can help parents to be ready to act on behalf of their child from the moment of birth.

For those who receive bad news, prenatal genetic testing also opens up another—though, for some, unacceptable—option: they could choose to terminate the pregnancy by having an elective abortion. Terminating a pregnancy is never an easy decision, even for those who are strongly "pro-choice" on the issue of abortion. People who have decided to end a much-wanted pregnancy often feel that they have no other option. This may be because they lack the emotional and financial resources to care for a child born with a serious illness, or that they are already physically drained by caring for another child with the same disorder, or because they are coping with any number of distressing life circumstances. Even people who are staunchly anti-abortion in theory have found themselves making the painful choice to end a pregnancy based on genetic test results. As one woman put it:

> It was a choice between terrible and awful. Watching a bright, alert, happy baby die is terrible and abortion is awful.

No outsider can determine for you whether this option to terminate a pregnancy is the right one. Its acceptability must emerge from the melting pot of your personal values and from the realities operating within your life. But it does exist as an option when prenatal genetic testing is used.

As you consider the balance of advantages and disadvantages of prenatal genetic testing, you should also think about the effects these tests can have on other family members, particularly on a family member who already has been diagnosed to have exactly the same genetic disorder that the test seeks to identify. What message might the prenatal test send? What would that child think if the parents chose to terminate the pregnancy to prevent the birth of another child with the very same genetic condition? One mother of a child with cystic fibrosis said that she could not consider prenatal testing at future pregnancies. She would not want her child to think that she didn't love him or give him reason to imagine that she had ever regretted he was born.

Genetic Tests to Determine Carrier Status

Carrier testing can be done at any point in a person's life. Finding out if you are a carrier of mutant genes associated with any one of a number of different genetic disorders doesn't seem at first to be terribly important. After all, what "carrier" means is that you have a mutant gene (and we all have several) but that it doesn't affect your health because there is another gene in the gene pair, one which is fully functional and can fulfill the body's needs quite adequately by itself. The mutant gene is, for all intents and purposes, medically invisible. No harm to health is done by its presence. So why bother to test for it?

Actually, there are times when knowing your carrier status might be useful, especially when you are planning to have children. As we have just seen in the section above on prenatal testing, exposing the hidden genes that parents carry can help identify the genetic illnesses for which the fetus is at higher risk. If both prospective parents happen to be carriers of the same flawed gene for a recessive disorder, then there is a 25 percent chance at each pregnancy that the child will inherit flawed genes from both parents and (since neither gene in the pair will then be functional) develop the disorder. If the flawed gene resides on the X chromosome, then a woman who is a carrier will, on average, pass that gene along to half of her sons. Because the partner chromosome to the X is the Y, and the Y chromosome doesn't contain functional genes that can mask mutant genes on the X, sons who inherit that mutant gene will develop the health problem associated with it. The knowledge of their own carrier status would permit such individuals and couples to be aware of the risk to their offspring and to then seek prenatal testing to determine the exact genetic situation for the fetus.

The decision about whether to pursue carrier testing is no different from any other genetic-testing decision. Once again, we can rely on the same four questions of our template to help us make a decision. And, of course, there are a few caveats specific to carrier testing that you will need to keep in mind.

It can be hard to know if a particular recessive gene is present in the family. Recessive genes can—and typically do—lie low for generations. They rarely reveal their presence. The main clue will generally come along in the form of a diagnosis of a genetic disorder for a person in the family, something that will seem to everyone like a bolt out of the blue. Once that happens, and the word spreads throughout the family network, then it becomes possible to get an estimate of what your risk is of being a carrier. A physician or genetic professional can use the rules of inheritance to calculate your risk based on your relationship to the person who has been diagnosed with the disorder. Another clue can be your connection to an ethnic or heritage group that has a higher frequency of the disorder. Here the known facts about the prevalence of particular disorders in different population groups can be used to provide you with a risk figure. For example, Caucasian individuals in the United States can be told that they have a 1/25 (or 4 percent) chance of being a carrier of a mutant gene associated with cystic fibrosis. African Americans who trace their family origins back to regions of the world where malaria was widespread can be told that they have a 1/10 (or 10 percent) chance of carrying the gene associated with sickle-cell anemia. Sometimes the frequency of carriers in a particular population is not known with any accuracy, and only a rough estimate can be given. These calculations or estimates can give you a ballpark figure for what your own risk is. You must evaluate that risk number for yourself to see if it is high enough— or if the disorder is serious enough—to warrant your attention.

Following guidelines recommended by the American College of Obstetricians and Gynecologists, expectant mothers are automatically offered carrier testing for certain genetic diseases. Testing for cystic fibrosis is relevant for women of European Caucasion ancestry, testing for Tay-Sachs disease is relevant for women of Ashkenazi Jewish ancestry, etc.

The genetic test can yield clear-cut information on your carrier status in several different situations:

- When a single mutation is known to occur (as for sickle-cell anemia and Tay-Sachs disease) or when a limited number of mutations are known to occur, the test can look directly for these to determine whether or not you are a carrier.
- The test can also look for the specific mutation that has been found in the genetic material of the family member with the disorder.
- The genetic test can detect particular mutations that have very distinctive characteristics, such as a chemical repeat that expands a small region of DNA into a longer one.

But not every genetic test result is definitive, and for some tests it will be hard to determine, with absolute certainty, if you are a carrier. An uncertainty arises when there are a large number of possible mutations in the target genes. Some of these mutations may be common while others may be quite rare, appearing only in very few families. Most carrier tests are designed to look for the common mutations. If you are told that you don't have any of the common mutations, it substantially reduces your risk of being a carrier, but it doesn't eliminate the risk completely. There remains a small chance that you could have one of the rare mutations that the test doesn't look for. Unless you know what mutation has already been found to be in your family, this is probably the best that carrier tests can do.

In contrast to prenatal genetic tests, which have a very restricted window of opportunity (the early months of gestation), carrier tests can be done at many different points in a person's life depending on the circumstances: prior to having children, at the point of having children, or after an affected child or sibling or relative is diagnosed. The wider choice for the timing may itself present something of a problem as people (such as Ted in the second vignette above) are left to figure out when is the right time. Should it be done before a person becomes sexually active? Should carrier testing be postponed until just before marriage—or before starting a family? Does it make any sense to have carrier testing if you are done having children or not planning to have any children? As we have seen in chapter 5, there are some wrong times for genetic testing. Because of all the emotional upheavals that it can evoke, genetic testing—including carrier testing—should not be attempted during especially stressful or difficult periods in one's life. And many professionals assert that carrier testing should never be done on children unless there is a definite health benefit (to the child) to be gained (see chapter 5). However, other professionals disagree. They offer the view that genetic information may be taken on board more easily by children when they are in their preteen years. As you can see, there are no hard-and-fast rules to go by. Ultimately, you must determine for yourself, given the reality of your own life, if the timing is likely to be suitable as you make your own carrier-testing decision.

When it comes to assessing the balance of advantages and disadvantages of having a genetic test that can reveal carrier status—the last area of the decision process—two items usually attract the most attention: the value of the information for the health of one's own future children, and the value of this information for others in the extended family. As we have seen, carrier testing of the parents can be a prelude to the use of prenatal genetic testing at future pregnancies, especially if the genetic status of the parents is such that it presents a risk for the development of health problems in their children.

Beyond the immediate family, who else is entitled to know about our personal genetic makeup? We share our genes with our relatives. As we discussed in chapter 4, it is generally held that there is a moral obligation to inform other family members of possible health risks as we become aware of them ourselves. For some families, this is routine and can easily be accomplished in the normal hubbub of family life. For others, the sharing of such information can be a difficult, if not an impossible, task because of such factors as distance or the toxic residue of past disagreements.

Genetic counselors and other genetic professionals are always willing to help, but the main initiative must come from the person who was tested. How fully this obligation to inform can be honored must be considered as part of the decision process.

At the same time, people have been reluctant to have carrier testing for fear that their information will go beyond the family and end up in the hands of prospective employers and insurance companies. People worry that the information could be used to deny them jobs or to raise their insurance premiums to unaffordable levels. The actual record about current misuse of carrier information is murky. In the past, misunderstandings about carrier status have indeed occurred when that information found its way into the wider community. For example, in the 1970s, when sickle-cell gene testing was first conducted, individuals who were found to be carriers (or said to have "sickle-cell trait") were often regarded, incorrectly, as having an actual illness by teachers, prospective employers, and insurance companies. Education was curtailed, jobs were lost, and insurance coverage was affected for many of these people.

Presymptomatic Genetic Tests

Presymptomatic genetic testing is the form of testing that can be done for a genetic disorder which is of the type that does not appear in childhood but, instead, develops later on in life. Although there are several other illnesses for which presymptomatic testing can be done, the poster child for this type of genetic disorder is Huntington disease. Huntington disease is brought on by a single mutant gene. Its effects (which start with loss of muscle control and balance) are not observed until a person is in his or her forties or fifties. In the past, the children of a person with Huntington disease would have no way of knowing if they had inherited the mutant gene until the first symptoms appeared. Often, by this time, they had had their own families, so that their children were now at risk too. After the mutant gene causing

Huntington disease was found, it became possible to use genetic testing to identify those individuals who have this gene long before the first symptoms appear. And such genetic testing can also provide relief to those at-risk individuals (with a parent having Huntington) who have not, in fact, inherited the mutant gene, and who can be informed, via genetic testing, that they will not develop the disease. With presymptomatic testing, a giant question mark hovering over people's lives can be removed.

Presymptomatic genetic testing differs in a significant way from the susceptibility-gene testing that has been the main subject of this book. The key element of presymptomatic testing is that the presence of the mutant gene is both necessary and sufficient for the disorder to occur. The test is definitive. It reveals whether or not the late-onset disorder will ever develop. If the mutant gene is found, the disorder will occur—although it may not happen until many years in the future. If the mutant gene is not found, the disease will not occur. In contrast to this, with susceptibility-gene testing, the situation is far more complicated because other genes, as well as environmental and lifestyle factors, contribute to the disease. The presence of a mutant susceptibility gene, by itself, is neither necessary nor sufficient for the disease to occur. As we have seen elsewhere in this book, if a susceptibility-gene test detects a mutant gene, it means that an individual's risk is increased. Although the probability of developing the disorder is higher than it is for someone without the mutant susceptibility gene, it is not definite that the individual will develop it. But with Huntington disease and other single-gene disorders of delayed onset, the presence of the gene is conclusive.

You should keep in mind a few special points as you ponder your decision about pursuing presymptomatic genetic testing. As always, the same four decision questions apply, and, naturally, your family health history is key to learning whether or not you are at risk for a disorder. With Huntington disease, myotonic muscular dystrophy, and other conditions for which presymptomatic genetic testing is possible, the disorder should already have appeared in the family before testing is considered. There will likely be strong indications that emerge from the family history pointing to the possibility that you may be at risk. It is important to be certain of the diagnosis afflicting the ill relative, and for this you should check with medical professionals who are expert in the disease. Other disorders can have some of the same symptoms and present with some of the same features. It will do no good to have genetic testing for the Huntington-disease mutation, for instance, if the real problem is another illness. Unless you are sure of the diagnosis, a genetic test showing that the characteristic Huntington mutation is absent would be falsely reassuring if the real culprit is another illness—an illness for which you might still be at risk.

People who have undergone presymptomatic genetic tests report that the wait for results can be an emotional roller-coaster from beginning to end. This emotional component is so marked that protocols (fixed procedures) have been established which are followed wherever the genetic testing is done. These protocols generally turn the testing into a multistep affair—involving several visits to physicians and genetic professionals with many opportunities for discussion and counseling—before the blood sample is collected. What this means is that anyone proceeding with testing should be prepared for a lengthy run-up to the actual testing.

Although the presymptomatic test for Huntington and similar diseases is almost always definitive, there are certain rare genetic circumstances for which the test results are ambiguous. This occurs for a few DNA signatures whose medical outcomes remain unclear. As more becomes known, these ambiguities will disappear.

As usual, even when the test definitively identifies the presence of the mutant gene, exactly when in the future the disorder may appear cannot be determined from genetic-test results.

The Huntington disease test was one of the first presymptomatic genetic tests to come into use in the medical setting. Since its availability in the mid-1980s, genetic professionals have gained considerable experience with it. There is a lot that has been learned, not the least of which has to do with the importance of timing. With presymptomatic testing, many people who decided to have testing did so before major life events such as getting married, having children, or embarking on the rigorous preparations for a job or career. And the same restrictions we have seen in chapter 5 about genetic testing of children also apply here. In a nutshell, parents cannot decide to have their children tested, because doing so would deny their children (such as Alexis in the third vignette at the start of this chapter) the right to decide for themselves. In fact, most of the people at risk for Huntington have decided against genetic testing. When children grow up and are capable of thinking this through, they and they alone can decide what personal genetic information they wish to have about themselves. There are times, however, when this rule is set aside. A major reason for doing so would be if there is some health benefit to the child from knowing. This is the case for disorders such as familial adenomatous polyposis (FAP), where early colonoscopy and removal of polyps or colon tissue are medical interventions effective in delaying or even preventing the onset of colon cancer. Here the benefit is clear. If there is no health benefit to be gained, then genetic testing of children for late-onset disorders must await the time that the child can decide for himself or herself.

A major factor in deciding about presymptomatic genetic tests seems to be one's views about uncertainty. For some people, removing the uncertainty hanging over their lives is a clear benefit. It eliminates the emotional distress associated with not knowing whether they will develop the disorder, and it gives them information that allows them to plan their lives with more assurance. If they are found not to have the mutant gene, they are able to cast off their worries and think more about a future uncomplicated by the disease. They can decide to have children without concern that they might be passing the mutant gene on to them. One young man summed it up: "You can't pass on what you don't have." He began to take steps to live out the normal course of his life free of worries about developing Huntington disease. If, on the other hand, the test reveals that the mutant gene is present, people can alter their life plans in the face of the anticipated future illness. They can arrange to do things like traveling earlier in their lives than they might have otherwise. They can seek prenatal testing to avoid passing on the gene to their children. And they can make plans to ensure proper care for themselves once the disorder arrives.

For others, there is a kind of comfort in *not* knowing. Not knowing brings with it a measure of hope that they might be spared and frees them from having to cope with the possibility of a test result that shows the disorder will eventually arrive. As one woman explained, "You can't unring a bell." Once the test result is given, that knowledge—and its impact on a person's life—is irreversible. And, of course, for both groups, those who choose testing and those who do not, the inevitable concerns about insurance coverage, should the test reveal the presence of the mutation, are also very much present.

Decision Aids

As consumers have done for the common disorders, those considering genetic testing for these less common disorders have often talked to others—doctors, family, and friends—as they worked toward their decision. Having such sympathetic and patient people to listen and help one think more clearly is certainly a plus. Sometimes, despite everyone's best intentions, these conversations are less than helpful. Those who are consulted may have an inadequate knowledge of the family dynamics, of the many facets of genetic testing, and of the rare disorders themselves to offer more than a sympathetic ear. Disappointingly, others may have their own personal agendas, strongly advocating testing just because a test happens to be available or rejecting testing with equal fervor because they feel it is at odds with their own personal beliefs, religious views, or social preferences.

Here too an important source of expertise that can help during the various stages of the decision process are the patient support groups. Consumers have found that contact—in person or via the computer—with people who have firsthand knowledge of the disorder and who have been on the same decision-making journey has gone a long way to help them clarify their own thoughts and come to closure. Ways to reach these organizations are included in this book's Resources section.

The tools of modern genetics are becoming very powerful, and genetic tests are increasingly being used in a number of different ways in the world of medical care. Tests, mandated by the state, are being carried out on newborns to identify genetic diseases, such as phenylketonuria (PKU), that can be treated immediately to prevent any mental or physical damage from occurring. And genetic tests are increasingly being used to decide which of the available medical treatments are likely to be the most effective, thereby tailoring—or personalizing—treatments to one's own genetic makeup. In these situations, our four-part decision-making apparatus points to the value of genetic testing because the benefits so clearly outweigh any possible harms, and time is usually of the essence in initiating treatments. Keeping newborns from suffering irreparable harm and employing treatments that are likely to be the most effective are all major goals of medicine. But for most other prenatal, carrier, presymptomatic, and susceptibility-gene testing situations, the decision may not be so clear and the hard work of personal decision making must be done.

CHAPTER NINE

The Future of Genetic Medicine

For decades we have seen how the astonishing advances made in genetics laboratories have steadily been introduced into medical practice. Techniques for probing into the worlds of embryos and fetuses—and uncovering some of the genetic secrets concealed there—have become standard procedures offered to pregnant women in the course of their prenatal care. Nowadays, newborn babies are tested for any of several genetic illnesses, so that treatments can be started early before harmful effects set in. And testing to establish the genetic status of adults with regard to single-gene disorders such as cystic fibrosis and Tay-Sachs disease is becoming fairly common. As a result, it seems inevitable that the discovery of susceptibility genes—genes that can help us know our individual predispositions to illness—will also have a strong impact on the world of health care, creating what many consider to be the new age of genetic medicine.

It is expected that in this new age, all of us will know our own genetic makeup and become attuned to any trouble spots in it. This knowledge of our vulnerabilities will open up a host of new opportunities, allowing us to practice prevention—to take steps ahead of time that may help to derail or diminish any disease process—and enabling us to live longer and healthier. We will be able to cast off the yoke of health problems that have afflicted past generations in our families. These new genetic tests will make it possible to have our medical care tailored to our individual genetic makeup, so that we will receive the most effective treatment available. Already some leading scientists have had their own DNA completely decoded. Companies are competing to find ways to bring down the costs so that it can be made more affordable for anyone to obtain his or her own complete genetic makeup. There are claims from leading researchers and health-care experts that genetic medicine is no longer a distant dream but is an emerging reality that will be a defining characteristic of twenty first century medicine. Perhaps.

But if the experience of the consumers and professionals who have contributed their experiences and wisdom to this book is any indication, then there are a number of significant obstacles that will have to be overcome if this new age of genetic medicine is going to enter beneficially into our lives. Let's take a look at what has to happen for genetic medicine to fulfill its promise of advancing our health and well-being.

Protections against Genetic Discrimination

By far, the biggest obstacle in the path of genetic medicine is the potential for the misuse of one's genetic information. Consumers are deeply concerned about this. They fear that any personal genetic information revealed in a genetic susceptibility test, rather than being helpful, might come back to haunt them. They fear that health-insurance providers, employers, and even the government itself will use this information to deny them the opportunities, services, and protections granted to others. These worries are not limited just to the consumers. Genetic and medical professionals share these concerns as well, and they feel an obligation to bring up the possibility of such discrimination when discussing genetic testing with their clients.

There are good reasons for all the concern about the possible misuse of genetic information. The suffering caused by past eugenics policies (see chapter 1, pp. 4–5) has not completely faded from public memory. Even without having detailed knowledge of that history, consumers are aware that genetic information has been used to punish people. Many of those interviewed in this study have had their own personal experiences of present-day discrimination—or have heard the stories circulating through their families. Coupled with reports in the media about insurance denied for genetic reasons and surreptitious genetic testing by employers, to many it seems a sure bet that genetic susceptibility tests will provide the raw material for new and painful forms of discrimination.

Consumers worry that if insurance companies learn of a genetic predisposition, their rates will go up or they will be denied coverage for illnesses that genetic tests identify as being more likely. They worry even more that their children, without actually being tested themselves, will be labeled as genetically compromised. The uninsurability problem might then be passed down from generation to generation, just like freckles or curly hair. In this anxiety-laden atmosphere, many have refused to undergo genetic testing.

The public's foreboding about genetic discrimination has not gone unnoticed. Most state governments have issued protective laws that promote patient privacy by restricting access to genetic information. These laws vary from state to state, but their intent is to enhance the confidentiality of genetic information. At the federal level, the Health Insurance Portability and Accountability Act of 1996 (HIPAA) offers some specific protections for those who are enrolled in group health plans. The Americans with Disabilities Act (ADA) has been interpreted to provide some protection against job discrimination for those found to have a genetic predisposition to illness. Many people are unaware of these laws. Others know about them but doubt their effectiveness. One agitated consumer felt that any promise of genetic privacy was "quaint"; that there would be no way in this computer age, with electronic medical records out in cyberspace, for such protections to be realistic.

On May 21, 2008, an important step was taken in the direction of firm national legal protection. After thirteen years of legislative foot-dragging, the Genetic Information Nondiscrimination Act (GINA) was signed into law, to take effect in late 2009. GINA prohibits health-insurance providers (for both group and individual policies) from requesting genetic information or from using genetic information to set premiums or to limit benefits. It prohibits employers from using genetic information in hiring, firing, or promotion. GINA thus covers health insurance and the workplace, two main areas of concern. It does not cover long-term-care insurance and disability insurance, and it does not cover people in the military.

It remains to be seen whether or not the prohibitions will actually work, or whether they will be circumvented in actual practice by insurance companies or employers. It will take time for consumers to see how well its provisions are understood and followed by insurers and employers, and to discover if loopholes exist. We can hope that GINA succeeds in guarding genetic privacy, preventing genetic discrimination, and permitting people to feel confident that their genetic information is secure and won't be abused.

A related problem needs attention. In contrast to most other businesses that seek to cultivate good interactions with their customers, the insurance industry has an unenviable reputation for being unfriendly, unhelpful, and unwilling to see their clients as anything other than potential cheats and threats to profit margins. "Insurance-company customer service" is regarded by many as an oxymoron. Far too many people know their health-insurance providers through what I am calling the "health-insurance hassle." This hassle begins with the apparently automatic rejection of valid claims, followed by the need for endless phone calls and letters to sort out matters. This hassle continues when consumers have to negotiate their way past stubborn "customer representatives" to find people qualified to understand the value of genetic testing and the preventative steps that can be taken if a mutation is found. And this hassle expands when consumers have to impose on their own physicians in order to enlist their aid in the battle for benefits. It is unlikely that any other business enterprise could stay afloat after putting its customers through such indignities. Genetic medicine will not be employed by many who need it and who would otherwise seek its benefits until this problem is addressed.

In an environment in which misuse of their genetic information is expected, it is not surprising that consumers seeking

genetic testing have adopted a number of strategies to try to protect themselves. Some of these self-protection strategies (paying
out of pocket, using false names, requesting the use of shadow
files, and the like) are more appropriate for plot lines in cloak-
and-dagger movies than for twenty-first-century high-tech medicine. These actions, products of near-desperation, raise a number
of red flags. Many genetic professionals assert that ultimately such
practices will do more harm than good. These practices, they say,
will only promote the stigma associated with genetic illness and
compromise the quality of medical care. Dr. Elizabeth Petty, professor of Internal Medicine and Human Genetics at the University
of Michigan, has put it this way: "People are worried about being
labeled that they are predisposed to a genetic disease. We perpetuate that by keeping it separate and saying, 'Yes, there is a problem
and we have to keep this secret.' I think that type of action fosters
that kind of thinking. What I tell patients—and what I believe is
true—is that we are all predisposed to various diseases. Some of us
have the opportunity to know what we are predisposed to because
there are tests out there to help us figure that out. But we are all
predisposed to something. We all have mutations. We are all
flawed in some way. The more we know about genetic backgrounds, the more helpful it may be for the medical profession
taking care of us, and for that reason the information should be in
the medical record."

   The perceived need for self-protections against insurance-
company discrimination has pushed some consumers a step farther.
They opt to completely exclude their medical doctors from the testing process by using the services of companies that provide direct-
to-consumer genetic testing. Needless to say, direct-to-consumer
testing has sparked some controversy. Some states permit it; others
prohibit it. Some have not yet taken a stand. Professional groups are
all of one mind: they find it unacceptable. The Board of Directors of
the American College of Medical Genetics has issued a policy
statement that includes the following: "[T]he self-ordering of
genetic tests by patients over the telephone or the Internet, and their

use of genetic 'home testing' kits, is potentially harmful. Potential harms include inappropriate test utilization, misinterpretation of test results, lack of necessary follow-up, and other adverse consequences." The Federal Trade Commission has issued a consumer advisory, "At Home Genetic Tests: A Healthy Dose of Skepticism May Be the Best Prescription," urging consumers to use great caution before embarking on any genetic testing done in this fashion.

But some consumers see merit in the self-testing option for susceptibility-gene testing. They find it a useful way to obtain genetic information while ensuring their privacy.

> Finally, we found a lab that . . . allows the patient to do the entire thing—confirm or rule out hemochromatosis—and basically diagnose yourself. That certainly is not very popular with the medical community. However, if it is the difference between doing the test or not doing the test, or a patient finding out if they have it or not, I would say it's important for them to find out. So, a person can order the testing themselves, get the results themselves. No one else gets the results or sees them.

Most other consumers who have worked with genetic counselors hold the opposite view. They feel that having access to the services of the medical community is crucial for understanding their real risk, for dealing with the emotional wallop of the test results, and for establishing the best possible program of surveillance or treatment.

> I think that, for me, even though I wanted to know my results right away, I think it's good having a time period when you think about it and a time when you go and you sit and talk with somebody about the results as they tell you the results. The day I got my results I was sitting with a genetic counselor. The next person who walked through the door was the gynecological oncologist. The next person who walked through the door was my gastroenterologist. So, I had a whole bunch of people there talking to me about what my specific screening recommendations are. There are general

recommendations, but you have to look at a pedigree to know what the specific recommendations should be for a person.

―――――――

With a situation like this you have to have some type of rapport with your health-care provider, whether it be the physician, the nurse practitioner, or the nurse in the office. It has to be someone who is well informed and you have some rapport with, and so much of the information that we communicate is as non-verbal language. . . . I like the Internet, I think it's a wonderful tool, but on some issues I think you really need that follow-up with a health-care provider who really knows you as a person.

―――――――

The Internet is wonderful, and it can also be dangerous. Sometimes too much information, when you are not able to handle it, can scare you to death. I think you need to sit down and talk with a human being who has training in the whole genetics picture. At times when we were going through counseling you felt like you were in Biology 101 again, but, after it was all done, it all made sense why they did the steps they did during the session.

The new era of genetic medicine must be built on a foundation free from harassment and from discrimination of any kind. It would indeed be unfortunate if the damaging practices of the past (and even of the present) are allowed to contaminate the future. Whether it is through robust legal actions or through better corporate practices, consumers must come to have confidence that their genetic privacy, and that of their families, will be protected and that they will always be treated with dignity and respect. The longer it takes for this to happen, the longer it will take genetic medicine to reach its full potential.

Better Genetic Training of the Medical Community

A number of the consumers interviewed in this study reported that their doctors—those providing patient care in offices, specialty centers, and hospitals—did not recognize the possibility of their higher hereditary risk even when the warning signs were there. Too many primary-care physicians and specialists are in the dark about the availability of genetic testing or the challenging human issues that accompany such testing. Frequently, consumer awareness of the existence of genetic tests came from newspapers, magazine stories, pamphlets, and from support-group programs, not from their own doctors. There are reasons for such a knowledge deficit in the medical community. The main one is that medical training often does not provide medical students with sufficient background in genetics. And then, once in practice, given the rapid pace of discovery, it is difficult for doctors to keep up with genetic advances and to make use of them.

> One reason, frankly, it's been difficult for me to get this arranged is just logistics. . . . I really wanted to have my own doctor do it, and that is very hard to do. Insurance doesn't want to pay; the lab didn't know how to do it. I actually had the blood drawn for it once, but they couldn't pull it off. My doctor had no idea and his office had no idea where I could get it done. So they ended up having to throw my blood away. They couldn't do it. Everybody seemed sort of clueless.

All too often, even when genetic tests were ordered, doctors were unable to interpret the results.

Promoting genetic expertise is not a frill. Genetics is already important. And it is becoming more and more so as genetic research delivers a wider array of susceptibility tests and also expands its presence in the areas of diagnosis and treatment. The advent of new "gene-chip" technologies may soon make it possible to carry out genetic testing for many different gene variations—associated with different disorders—all at the same time. In the area of treatment, a new genetic-medicine specialty known as pharmacogenomics is emerging. It is based on the search for small variations in genes that indicate how effectively one's body can respond to specific drugs in fighting illness. For someone with an illness, a particular drug may be effective only if that person possesses certain specific gene variations. This same drug may work less effectively, or it may not work at all, in people who lack these specific gene variations. Genetic testing to determine the presence or absence of these gene variations can be used to decide which drug or which treatment option would be most effective. This can spare patients wasting time with ineffective treatments, and it can allow their doctors to recommend right away the treatments that are most likely to work. Doctors will need to be able to use this type of genetic knowledge in their everyday practices. So, whether as a means of identifying those at higher risk for a particular disorder, or as a means of selecting the most effective treatment for those with a disorder, genetics is simply too important for health-care professionals to ignore.

For medical care to incorporate genetic knowledge and for consumers to receive its benefits, it is critical that genetics as a subject play a larger part in medical education than it currently does. Unquestionably, it is difficult to add material into an already bulging medical curriculum. But it will have to be done. For doctors already in practice, there will have to be continuing-education mechanisms that provide the requisite background. However it is accomplished, it is crucial that health-care practitioners take family histories and recognize patterns of illness in families. It is essential that they become knowledgeable about the full spectrum of human issues related to genetic testing, so that they can assist their patients in thinking through whether genetic testing is appropriate for them. In an age of genetic medicine, there is no alternative.

Beyond better genetics education for physicians, there are other issues that the medical community needs to address. Because there are only a limited number of genetic professionals (including genetic counselors), it is likely that more and more genetic-testing decisions will be made with the help of one's own doctor during an office visit. Physicians are under enormous time pressure. The typical office visit does not allow enough time for most genetic matters to be introduced and adequately discussed. The usual physician/patient interaction is simply too short for presenting the genetic-testing option along with the educational and decision making tools that are required. There is a clear need for the preparation of a new range of educational materials and decision aids. These should be made available in doctors' offices to supplement the normal verbal exchange of the visit. Patients have different learning styles and widely varying degrees of familiarity with scientific concepts. A variety of resources—printed, video, computer based—will be required to meet their needs.

In addition to such new educational approaches, members of the medical community must be committed to support and accompany their patients on what can be a lengthy decision-making journey. All too often, people in this study felt that their doctors left them without adequate assistance as they tried to learn, consider, and decide:

> When you are doing this, you are kind of on your own. There has not been any guidance. The whole process, it's just been very confusing to me.

Support groups and others can be extremely helpful. But surely physicians, as well as other members of the medical community who meet with patients in the course of their office visits, have a professional obligation to create an infrastructure that assures that there really is meaningful understanding of the benefits and burdens offered by genetic medicine. At every stage, the options made available by genetic medicine should be accompanied by an informed decision process. This can be done—and done well.

> This is the most important thing, I think, for our generation. That my doctors take it seriously when I ask a question and they treat me seriously in terms of my questions. They explain things scientifically; they ask me questions to make sure I have understood

what they have said; and I ask them questions. And that included all of the genetic information. That is why I am still alive. It's because my doctors took that time.

This obligation doesn't end with the decision itself. There should be procedures in place to follow up with that person—over months, maybe even years—as the consequences of the decision are felt. Since physician time is so limited, then others—especially nurse-specialists in cancer clinics and other staff members who are part of the health-care team—will need to be trained to step in and help. Facilitating the decision process surrounding the new genetic susceptibility tests is as important as working in the laboratory to develop them.

There Are Also Individual Responsibilities

The era of genetic medicine has implications for each of us. With its emphasis on prevention, genetic medicine requires us to become proactive guardians of our own health. To actually receive the benefits, we have to take on a number of responsibilities.

- We have to be aware of our family health history by gathering the information and organizing it in an accessible way.
- We have to make our family health histories available to all of our health-care providers and to update them as the information changes.
- We have to think through for ourselves the advisability and acceptability of genetic testing, using the four questions described in this book as a guide.
- We have to check back periodically with our health-care providers to find out if any of the genetic or medical information has changed, to see if there are new findings regarding those variants of unknown significance and new modes of prevention, or to discuss any reports in the media or on the Internet that raise questions in our minds.

- Whether or not we choose to have genetic testing, we should establish a personal health-maintenance plan in consultation with our health-care providers—one that reflects our individual circumstances and preferences. Such a plan should be developed to keep us in the best of current health, to set monitoring targets so that any problems are noted early, and, if illness occurs, to allow us to explore the options and select the types of treatments that are likely to do us the most good. Michael Retsky, co-founder and board member of the Colon Cancer Alliance, has noted that "when you buy a new car, you get a maintenance schedule that comes with it. There is nothing like that in health care that says this is what you should be doing for the next five years. There is nothing like that out there. There should be."

One more thing. We must be prepared, as individuals and as citizens, to contribute to discussions and decisions that will determine the future of genetic medicine. We have to work together—through support groups or through our elected representatives or through participation in public meetings of government panels—to confront the problems and the many challenging questions that will surely arise.

A number of challenges are already upon us. It is clear to genetic professionals that members of many ethnic and heritage groups are underrepresented in their practices. How can we avoid creating a group of "have-nots" who are denied the opportunities for disease prevention? What are the best ways to ensure proper oversight of genetic tests, and access to these tests? How can we expand newborn genetic screening so that all children are protected equally? There are a number of new challenges waiting in the wings. With the increasing use of gene chips—or the advent of complete DNA sequencing, whenever that becomes affordable—the amount of genetic information to which we will have access will be daunting. How should these technologies be used? How will people be able to choose which information they would like to have—and which they would like to avoid? Should there be tests for genes associated with characteristics that are not clearly health related (height, hair color, "intelligence", "personality", etc.)? Of what value is such genetic information, and should it be sought under the banner of health care?

One way or another, the age of genetic medicine will unfold in the coming years. Whether it brings a bounty of good health and not the burden of genetic labeling, whether it is available to all and not just a few, whether we address the controversial questions that arise and deal with them properly is up to us. These issues will require our collective wisdom. If genetic medicine is to succeed, we must all be involved.

Appendix
A Brief Introduction to Genetics

What genes really are and what they actually do is quite different from what popular ideas sometimes suggest. This tutorial will provide a basic introduction to genetics. The goal is not to turn the reader into a research scientist but, instead, to show, with as few frills as possible, how it is that genes are sometimes connected with specific illnesses and the way those genes may be passed on in a family from one generation to the next. We will also see how tests can be done to find out about a person's specific genetic makeup. There are ten basic points in all.

Point 1: Genes Are Located on Chromosomes

Scientists are not yet certain how many *genes* we humans have. Estimates run from as few as 20,000 to as many as 100,000 different genes. Most current estimates favor the lower end of this range. Regardless of the actual number, all of our genes are repeated trillions of times throughout our body. They are found in every one of our body's cells. The *cell* is the building block that makes up all living organisms. Some organisms found in nature are amazingly small and simple—only one cell in size. Humans, however, are considerably larger. The human body is composed of trillions of cells, almost all of them highly specialized into different cell types such as muscle, nerve, blood, brain, and skin cells. These cell types are organized into groups to form organs and organ systems. All of these systems need to function in harmony for the whole body to operate smoothly. To make this happen, a multitude of different tasks—involving growth, repairing damage, coordinating with other parts of the body, and responding to the environment—must be carried out successfully by each of the cells in the body.

A gene is a unit that contains the instructions for how a cell should carry out a specific task. These genes are not floating about individually, but are connected in long ribbonlike or barlike structures called *chromosomes*. Chromosomes are all stored together in one portion of a cell, in a compartment called the *nucleus*.

Every species has a characteristic number of chromosomes. The number for corn is 20, for wheat, 42. In the frog the chromosome number is 26. In the mouse it is 40, and in the dog, 78. In humans the chromosome number is 46. This full complement of 46 is made up of 23 pairs of chromosomes.

Every human cell contains the same chromosome number, 46, except for two very special types of cells: egg cells in women and sperm cells in men. These cells contain 23 chromosomes. Each set of 23 contains one representative of every pair. When a sperm cell fuses with an egg cell to begin the chain of events that can lead to a new individual, the standard human chromosome number of 46 is restored.

To help distinguish one pair of chromosomes from another, scientists labeled the pairs of chromosomes with numbers from 1 through 22. The chromosome pairs from 1 through 22 are called the *autosomes*. The two members of each pair of autosomes are alike in size, shape, and the pattern of bands that appears after they are stained with special dyes in the laboratory. The *sex chromosomes* form the 23rd pair. This is the only pair in which the two members may be different in structure. In females, the pair is comprised of two large-sized chromosomes called "X" chromosomes. In males, the sex-chromosome pair has one X chromosome and a smaller chromosome, known as the "Y" chromosome, as the second member of the pair. Thus, for the pair of sex chromosomes, females are XX and males are XY.

All of the genes needed throughout the lifespan of an individual—from the fertilized egg to the adult—are stored on the chromosomes. Because there are 23 pairs of human chromosomes but thousands of human genes, it is clear that each chromosome contains many genes. Only the Y chromosome is gene-poor. Current evidence suggests that the Y chromosome contains only a few dozen genes.

Point 2: Chromosomes—and So Also Genes—Are Made Up of a Chemical Substance Called DNA

Chromosomes are made up of a very special type of molecule called DNA. (The letters stand for the full chemical name: deoxyribonucleic acid.) DNA is a very thin and a very long molecule. As is shown in figure A.1, each chromosome is actually a single, long, tangled thread of DNA. If the DNA in chromosome 1 (the largest chromosome) were to be untangled and stretched out (like the straightened string from an unraveled ball of yarn), it would measure about 20 inches in length. But in its normal tangled state within the microscopic nucleus of a human cell, the DNA thread occupies a vastly smaller space.

DNA is the genetic material. It is the chemical substance of which all genes are composed. The first glimpses into the nature of DNA came in 1953 and, by now, its structure is known in considerable detail. A sketch of the DNA molecule is shown in figure A.1. The DNA thread contains two strands that twist around each other in a spiral fashion, giving it the distinctive shape of a double helix.

The key components of each DNA strand are clusters of atoms, known as *bases*. There are four types of bases in DNA. These are adenine (A), guanine (G), thymine (T), and cytosine (C). Each of these bases is usually referred to just by its initial. Between each base on one strand and the corresponding base on the opposite strand is a chemical connection or bond. These chemical connections hold the two strands together. These connections are precise in that an A base in one strand can connect only with a T in the opposite strand, and a G can bond only with a C.

A gene is a section of DNA along the length of a chromosome. The section of DNA corresponding to each gene possesses a specific *sequence* of bases that determines the specific function of the gene. Genes vary in size. Some are small, occupying a very short section of the DNA thread. Others are very large, extending a considerable distance along the DNA. We can imagine each of the chromosomes as a cookbook containing hundreds or even thousands of individual recipes (some brief, some lengthy), all bound together, one following the next. In a cookbook, recipes of the same type—appetizers, salads, main

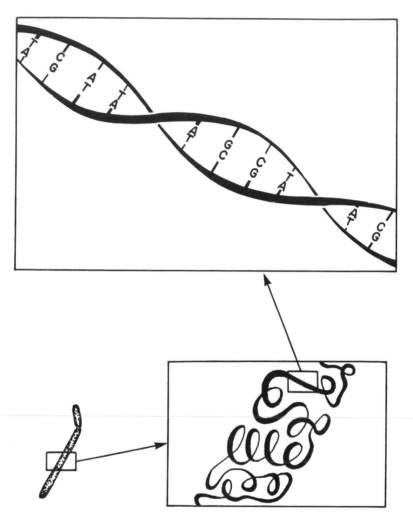

Figure A.1. A diagram representing magnified views of a chromosome's structure. The chromosome is at the lower left. A magnified portion of the chromosome (the section in the small rectangle) reveals that it consists of a long thread, the DNA molecule. A magnified portion of the DNA molecule (large rectangle at the top) shows that the thread consists of two strands that are held together by A-T and G-C bonds. The two strands twist around each other in a double helix.

dishes, desserts—are grouped into their own separate chapters. But on a chromosome, the genetic information is largely a jumble of different types of instructions for different types of tasks. A gene that helps a muscle contract might be located between a gene responsible for the early development of the digestive system and a gene involved in eye color.

And unlike a cookbook, which has few blank pages, each chromosome contains long stretches of DNA that do not seem to have any function. These long stretches may contain scraps of genes left over from our evolutionary past, antique recipes for functions that we no longer use. These regions may also contain the remains of viruses that infected our ancestors in eons past and inserted tiny bits of genetic material into chromosomes where they now lie abandoned. Some of these regions may also have useful functions that we do not yet understand.

Point 3: Genes Work Mostly by Producing Proteins

How can a gene, which is just a length of DNA along a chromosome, affect the activities of an organism? It can do this because the specific order, or sequence, of the bases (the A's, G's, T's, and C's) provides the code or recipe for making a specific *protein*. Proteins are cell substances that are composed of smaller subunits (called *amino acids*) connected together in a linear fashion. Within the nucleus of the cell, a complex set of operations is initiated. The instructions provided by the sequence of bases help the cell direct the assembly of a corresponding sequence of amino acids into a protein. In this way, a gene is responsible for producing its own particular protein.

Most of the life-supporting work of living organisms is carried out by proteins. There are different kinds of proteins with different types of functions. *Enzyme proteins* (better known just as "enzymes") act as catalysts, speeding up chemical reactions and allowing critical life functions such as digestion, growth, excretion, and response to the environment to take place rapidly and efficiently. *Structural proteins* are responsible for building the various parts of our body's architecture. The many components that we can see (such as bones, hair, and nails) which shape and give support to our bodies, as well as ones that can be seen only with the aid of a microscope (such as membranes surrounding cells or small particles within cells), contain proteins. *Regulatory proteins* coordinate different chemical processes that need to occur in a synchronized fashion. In these and in many other ways, proteins are central in all the biological functions necessary to sustain life.

Although every cell of an individual contains the same genes, the array of proteins produced in different types of cells is not the same. Each specific type of cell—whether it is from muscle, nerve, skin, liver, and so on—results from the presence of a specific mix of proteins. So in muscle cells, proteins are produced that are necessary for the muscle to contract. But a muscle cell does not produce proteins that are required for vision. Red blood cells produce those proteins necessary to transport oxygen around the body, but they don't produce any of the proteins involved in digestion. Our body cells, with their multitude of different proteins, provide the dynamic framework that makes life possible.

Despite the substantial influence that genes have on bodily activities, we should keep in mind that genes are not the only determining factors. The effects that genes have on our health are greatly influenced by the environment in which they function. This environment can be as local as the internal conditions of a cell, as temporary as the intrauterine world of the developing fetus, or as enormous as the vast array of external physical, chemical, cultural, and lifestyle factors that constitute the larger world in which we live. Sometimes the environmental impact is subtle, mildly altering the way a gene works or the effect that its presence ultimately has on the individual. Other times, the environmental influences can be substantial and decisive, completely camouflaging the presence of certain genes or intensifying the action of others.

Point 4: Genes (Nearly Always) Come in Pairs

The two chromosomes in any given pair contain the same set of genes and in the same order. Suppose a gene for a particular enzyme occurs at a certain position on one chromosome of the pair. The gene for that same enzyme will be found on the other chromosome at exactly the same position. We say that this gene occurs at the same location, or *locus*, on both members of the chromosome pair. This means that there are two copies of every gene in each cell of the body.

The only exception to this rule is the XY sex-chromosome pair in males. The X and Y chromosomes differ substantially in gene content The X chromosome contains many genes for many different types of activities. The Y chromosome has only a few genes. They are primarily involved in the development of the male reproductive system. As a result, males have only one copy of each X chromosome gene. Females, because their sex chromosome pair contains two X chromosomes, have two copies of each X chromosome gene.

Point 5: Members of a Pair of Genes Can Differ from Each Other

The two genes at the same locus (one on each chromosome in the chromosome pair) can be identical. That is, they can both have the same sequence of bases. When this occurs, both genes provide identical information for producing their specific protein product. However, the two genes do not have to be identical, and very often they are not. Genes at the same locus can have somewhat different DNA sequences. When this occurs, two somewhat different proteins can be produced under the direction of the genes in the gene pair.

Any change, variation, or (if it causes any type of problem) flaw in the standard or usual base sequence of a gene is called a *mutation*. A mutation can affect how a particular cell (and all cells that are formed from it) functions. Mutations can arise in many ways. They can arise in genes located in any of the cells of the body through accidents during cell division or exposure to DNA-damaging agents such as ultraviolet radiation from the sun, X-rays from medical tests, free radicals that form from chemical processes in the cells, or chemicals from the environment. Such mutations are not passed on to children. Only the individual in whom the mutation has occurred may suffer any harmful effects related to those changes in the DNA.

Mutations can also arise when mistakes occur in the DNA base sequence as new DNA is being made in sperm or egg cells. Such mutations can be passed on, through the fertilized egg, to children in the next generation and possibly to following generations.

Mutations or changes in a gene can alter the protein that is made. Some changes in the gene's base sequence will have only minor effects. The protein product may be slightly altered, but it will still work perfectly well. Other changes can have significant effects. This can happen when the altered protein product is so damaged that it works poorly or when the change results in no protein being made at all.

Point 6: Changes in Genes Can Sometimes Lead to Health Problems

Medical disorders result from the presence of mutations that interfere with gene function.

The term "single-gene disorders" refers to those medical conditions that arise when one or both of the members of a particular gene pair are unable to do their job properly. Even if all the other thousands of genes are doing their jobs well, the failure of just one gene pair, especially if that pair is responsible for a key activity, can have a harmful effect on how the whole body functions. This brings on health problems that can be extremely serious, even life threatening.

If a mutation or flaw in just one gene of the pair shows up in the form of a noticeable health problem, the gene mutation is called *dominant.* Myotonic muscular dystrophy, Huntington disease, and some forms of retinitis pigmentosa are examples of dominant disorders. In contrast to this, a *recessive* mutation is one that shows up as a health problem only when both genes of the pair have a mutation that interferes with their function. Spinal muscular atrophy, sickle-cell anemia, and cystic fibrosis are examples of recessive disorders. (Single-gene disorders are discussed in chapter 8 of this book.)

When a mutation is present, it may not be possible to predict precisely what its effect on health will be, either at the time of birth or later on as the individual develops and matures. Different mutations in the same gene can have different effects on health—from being almost unnoticeable to causing severe problems. Even the same mutation can affect different people differently. For instance, a tiny change in one of the genes responsible for making part of the hemoglobin molecule in our red blood cells can, in one person, result in a severe life-threatening form of sickle-cell anemia. Someone else, with exactly the same genetic mutation, can have a much milder case.

In contrast to the single-gene disorders are the "complex disorders." Many basic body functions are carried out by several different genes that interact with environmental factors (such as exposure to radiation, chemicals, and infections, as well as lifestyle habits such as diet, exercise, and smoking) in a complicated way that is still poorly understood. Complex disorders (the word "multifactorial" is also used) is the name given to those medical conditions that occur if there is some inadequacy in the function of one or more of those genes or if there is a less-than-optimal interaction between genes and environment. Here, the presence of a particular gene mutation may predispose those individuals to an illness that develops later in life but does not make the illness inevitable. Cancer, heart disease, diabetes, and many other common health problems fall into this category. (This is the type of disorder that is the major focus of this book.)

No one has a perfect collection of genes. All of us have some mutations in our DNA. It is estimated that each of us has about ten genes in which changes have occurred that could severely impair our health if they showed up. Fortunately, a change in our DNA does not always show up as a health problem. Whether a genetic disorder ever arises can depend on where the gene is located, whether the changes are dominant or recessive, and the type of task that the gene helps direct. For the complex disorders, it also depends on how important a role that gene actually has in whatever process it is involved, as well as the kinds of influence exerted by the environment.

Point 7: "Single-Gene" Disorders Show Different Patterns of Inheritance in Families

People have long sought ways to make sense of the patterns of inheritance they were observing in their families. With the groundbreaking experiments of the nineteenth-century Austrian monk Gregor Mendel and innumerable studies carried out around the world since that time, it has been possible to identify several patterns of inheritance exhibited by single genes. These patterns make it possible to understand the way that certain disorders can be passed through generations. Key features of these patterns are summarized in table A.1, which should be a useful guide to refer to while reading this discussion. Though our emphasis here is on genetic disorders, these same patterns underlie the inheritance of other typical human traits, such as hair type and blood type.

The Autosomal Dominant Pattern

If a dominant mutation occurs within a gene located on one of the 22 pairs of autosomes, it is called an *autosomal dominant* mutation. An illness caused by an autosomal dominant mutant gene can show up in successive generations of a family. Most often, a person with the illness is an individual who has a mutant gene along with the standard—or "normal"—gene. Such an individual will produce two different types of eggs (if female) or sperm (if male). Half of the eggs or sperm will have a set of 23 chromosomes that includes the chromosome with the normal gene; half of the eggs or sperm will have a set of 23 chromosomes that includes the chromosome with the flawed (mutant) gene. Half of the time, a fertilized egg produced at conception will receive (by chance) the normal gene. Half of the time, a fertilized egg will receive (by chance) the mutant gene. This means that a dominant mutant gene has a 50 percent chance of being passed from parent to child, where its presence will be evident. In the case of autosomal dominant disorders, males and females have an equal chance of inheriting the mutant gene and developing the disorder. Individuals in the family who do not have the disorder have no flawed genes to pass on, and so the disorder cannot show up in their children.

A Note on Probability

In small families, one cannot expect to observe a strict 50–50 pattern of autosomal dominant inheritance. The 50 percent chance of any given child inheriting the mutant gene is, it must be emphasized, a *probability*. It means that if 1,000 families in this situation (one parent with an autosomal dominant mutation) have 2,000 children, then about 1,000 of the children will inherit the gene and develop the disorder. It can happen, in

Table A.1. Patterns of Inheritance for Single-Gene Disorders

Type of Disorder	Parents	Children
Autosomal dominant	One has the flawed gene, and has (or will have) the disorder.	Each child has a 50% chance of inheriting the flawed gene, and thus a 50% chance of developing the disorder.
Autosomal recessive	One parent is a carrier, the other is not. Neither has the disorder.	No child will develop the disorder, though each has a 50% chance of carrying the flawed gene.
Autosomal recessive	Both parents are carriers. Neither will develop the disorder, though each has one copy of the flawed gene.	Each child has a 25% chance of not receiving a flawed gene. Such a child will not develop the disorder, and is also not a carrier. Each child has a 50% chance of receiving one copy of the flawed gene. Such a child will not develop the disorder, but is a carrier (like both parents). Each child has a 25% chance of having two copies of the flawed gene. Such a child will develop the disorder.
X-linked recessive	One of the mother's X chromosomes contains the flawed gene. She is a carrier but will not develop the disease, since the gene on her other X chromosome overrides it.	No daughters (XX) will develop the disorder, but each has a 50% chance of being a carrier (like her mother). Each son (XY) has a 50% chance of inheriting the flawed gene, and thus of developing the disorder because the Y chromosome has no corresponding gene to mask it.

a specific family with two or three children, that all of the children inherit the mutant gene. It can happen that none do. It can happen that the individuals with the disorder in one family are all males, or all females. Each fusion of sperm and egg is a separate, independent, chance event. The joining together of parental genes in each new child is independent of whatever may have occurred before in the family. Having one child with the disorder (or one child without the disorder) does not change the odds for the next child. The probability remains 50 percent.

The rule to remember is this: *The odds are the same at each pregnancy.*

The Autosomal Recessive Pattern

If a recessive mutation has occurred in a gene located on one of the 22 pairs of autosomes, it is called an *autosomal recessive* mutation. In contrast to a dominant mutation, a *recessive* mutation is one that shows up as a health problem only when both members of the gene pair are mutated.

As an example, let us suppose that we are looking at a gene pair that contains the instructions for making a particular enzyme. Let's suppose that this enzyme is responsible for catalyzing a reaction needed to produce an important cell substance. If an individual has a gene pair with one standard gene (a gene with instructions for making a properly functioning enzyme) and one mutant recessive gene (a gene that leads to an impaired nonfunctioning enzyme), there will be no health problems related to that enzyme. The amount of enzyme produced under the direction of the one functional gene is sufficient to ensure that enough of that cell substance is produced to meet the cell's needs. This means that even when only one gene of the pair is working correctly, enough normal protein is made for each cell to carry out the corresponding task. A person with this genetic makeup, who has one standard gene and one mutant recessive gene, is called a *carrier*. It is important to emphasize that carriers are healthy. Carriers do not suffer any ill effects from having the recessive mutant gene. In fact, most carriers have no idea that they have the mutant gene. Remember, we all carry several recessive mutant genes. The fact is that we usually do not know about them, because they are masked by the presence of a functional gene on the other chromosome.

Recessive mutant genes may lead to disorders in children when both parents are carriers. It is then possible for two mutant genes, one contributed by each parent, to come together when an egg is fertilized. Each carrier parent produces two types of egg or sperm. One type will have the chromosome with the normal gene; the other will have the mutant gene. When both parents are carriers, there is a one in four chance (or 25%) that an egg and a sperm each containing the mutant gene will join with each other to form the fertilized egg. When this happens, both genes of the pair (in the child) will be mutant genes. In our enzyme-production example, all of the enzyme protein produced by the pair of flawed mutant genes will be defective. With only defective protein present, the vital cell substance will not be produced. The health of individual cells and of the person with these genes will be impaired. Carrier parents can also have children who are carriers like themselves (one gene of the pair is flawed), and they can also have children who do not have the mutant gene (neither gene of the pair is flawed). At each pregnancy then, the probability is 25 percent for having a child with the disorder, 50 percent for having a healthy child who is a carrier, and 25 percent for having a healthy child who is not a carrier.

Because its presence is masked by the functionally normal gene, an autosomal recessive mutant gene can remain hidden for many generations. It is only when partners come together who happen to have, by chance, the same recessive mutant gene that there is a possibility (25 percent at each pregnancy) that the disorder will show up. For this reason, genetic disorders brought on by autosomal recessive genes tend to show up unexpectedly. Often, no one in the family can recall any illness like it having occurred before. But when such an illness does occur, this is a signal that other children in the same family may be carriers, as may cousins, aunts, uncles, and grandparents. For autosomal recessive disorders, males or females are equally likely to be affected.

As stressed above, it should *not* be expected that any particular family will have a distribution of inheritance that is the same as the average distribution of 25 percent (no mutant gene)/50 percent (carriers)/25 percent (showing the disorder). There is no requirement that one child in a family of four has to have the genetic illness. There is no guarantee that having one child with the illness means that the next three will be healthy. And it is not true that having several healthy children means that the next child is due to develop the illness. Sometimes more than one child in a family may inherit the double-recessive combination. Sometimes none of them will. Geneticists are fond of saying that "chance has no memory." This is their way of reminding people that two carrier parents face the same odds at every pregnancy.

The X-linked Patterns of Inheritance

Mutations on the X chromosome produce a different pattern of inheritance. All genes that are on the X chromosome are said to be X-linked. Males have only one X chromosome and thus males have only one copy of each of their X-linked genes. It turns out that one copy is enough to provide sufficient amounts of protein to meet cell needs. However, if any gene on the X chromosome of a male contains a mutation, there will be no second copy of the gene to rely on. There is no corresponding working gene on the Y chromosome that can mask it. This means that the disorder associated with the mutant gene will show up. For example, if there is a mutation in a male's X-chromosome gene for the muscle protein called dystrophin, it will show up as Duchenne muscular dystrophy, a disorder in which muscles deteriorate. If there is a mutation in a male's X-chromosome gene for a certain protein required for blood to clot when there is an injury, it will show up as hemophilia. Females who are carriers of these flawed genes generally show no sign of the disorder. They usually have, as part of their sex chromosome pair, a second X chromosome with a functional gene. This means that X-linked recessive mutations show up much more commonly in males.

A woman who is a carrier of an X-linked gene mutation will produce two different types of eggs. Approximately half will have the X chromosome with the normal gene, approximately half will have the X chromosome with the mutant gene. If an egg cell bearing the mutant gene is fertilized by a sperm cell bearing a Y chromosome, there will be no way to mask the presence of the mutant gene and its effects will show up in that male child. If an egg cell with the mutant gene is fertilized by a sperm cell with an X chromosome (with the normal gene), the resulting female child will be healthy and a carrier like her mother.

On average, *X-linked recessive* disorders are expected to appear in half of the male offspring of a woman who is a carrier. The other half, those males who had received from her the X chromosome with the functional gene, will be free of the disorder. Each pregnancy, of course, is a new toss of the genetic dice—it is not influenced by what has happened before in the family. Of her daughters, on average, half will be expected to be carriers like herself, and half will be expected to have received two copies of the normal gene. None of the daughters will have the disorder. When X-linked recessive mutant genes show up in males in two or more different places in a family, the affected relatives are all related to one another by females who are carriers. X-linked recessive disorders can also appear to "skip" one or more generations, as the gene is passed down through females who are carriers of the recessive mutation. The only way a female can have an X-linked recessive disorder is if her father has that disorder and her mother is a carrier of the mutant gene for that disorder. This can happen when an X-linked mutation occurs fairly often in the population, as is the case for the mutation that leads to colorblindness.

Frequently, an X-linked recessive disorder appears in a family in which there is no previous history of the disorder. Its sudden appearance can be explained in one of two ways. The mutant gene may have been present for generations, passed along by carrier females who were completely unaware of its presence. By chance, the chromosome bearing the mutant gene had never been paired with a Y chromosome. Or it may be that a brand new mutation has occurred. Geneticists have estimated that one in three new cases of an X-linked disorder are the result of such a new mutation. In the case of a new mutation, the mother of the boy with the genetic illness is not a carrier.

X-linked dominant mutations are very rare. When they occur, they show up in both males and females. If a man has a disorder brought on by such a mutation, all his daughters (who must have inherited his X chromosome to develop as females) will have the disorder. All of his sons (who must have inherited his Y chromosome) will be unaffected. If a female has an X-linked dominant mutation, she has the disorder and there is a 50 percent chance that each of her children, sons and daughters, will inherit the same disorder.

Point 8: Inheritance Patterns for the "Complex" (or "Multifactorial") Disorders Are Harder to Discern

Most of the common (and life-threatening) disorders that afflict people as they grow older—including heart disease, cancer, diabetes, and Alzheimer's disease—are not the result of defects in a single gene pair. They are the result of a breakdown in teamwork involving several different types of genes, along with influences from a variety of different environmental factors. Sometimes a flaw in one or more of the genes on the team will, over a long period of time, bring about the onset of symptoms. Sometimes it is environmental factors (diet or smoking or exposure to toxic substances or radiation) that serve as the actual trigger for the onset of illness. And sometimes, the finger of blame can be pointed at a complicated—and, unfortunately, still poorly understood—interaction among all the genetic and environmental factors. Thus the presence of a mutant gene does not ensure the onset of symptoms, but it makes an individual more likely, or susceptible, to developing them. Hence the term "susceptibility gene" is frequently applied to those genes which, when bearing mutations, increase the risk of developing very common health problems later on in life. Conversely, the absence of a mutant susceptibility gene does not prevent the disorder from ever making an appearance. The designations "complex" (because it is complicated) and "multifactorial" (because there is a mix of genetic and environmental factors) are certainly apt ways to describe the source of these common health problems. For cancer, current medical and scientific experience shows that inherited mutant susceptibility genes are involved only about 10% of the time.

For complex disorders, the general patterns of inheritance are not as straightforward as for single-gene disorders (table A.1). When trying to determine whether susceptibility genes are present, one must look at the family health history for a number of suggestive signs. The main signs are multiple occurrences (three or more) of the same disorder among individuals who are blood relations; the appearance of the disorder at an earlier age than is usual; and, in the case of cancer, primary tumors occurring more than once in the same person.

Even when they don't reveal themselves, mutant susceptibility genes can be passed along from parent to child just as are other genes.

Among the known susceptibility genes, those connected to breast/ovarian cancer and colon cancer follow an autosomal dominant inheritance pattern. There is a 50 percent chance at each pregnancy that the mutant gene will be passed on from the parent to the child (male or female). Those who inherit the mutant susceptibility gene have a higher risk of developing the disorder. Some susceptibility genes, such as those associated with hereditary hemochromatosis, follow a pattern akin to that of autosomal recessive inheritance. In this case, both parents must be carriers of a mutant susceptibility gene for there to be a 25 percent chance at each pregnancy that both mutant genes will be passed on to the child, raising the risk that the disorder will appear. Still another known susceptibility gene, that for Alzheimer's disease, raises the risk for developing the disease when in single or double dose. The risk is higher if an individual has inherited a double dose of the mutant susceptibility gene.

Point 9: There Are Different Types of Tests That Reveal One's Genetic Status

Today the study of human genes is one of the most active areas in medical research. Scientists are learning a great deal about how changes in the genetic material can lead to various health problems. Once this relationship is understood, tests that look for the genetic changes underlying these problems become possible. The three main types of techniques that are used are microscope-based techniques, biochemical techniques, and techniques that are capable of probing the genetic material, DNA, itself.

Microscope-based Tests

Some disorders result from an incorrect number of chromosomes (above or below the normal total of 46). Best known among such chromosomal disorders is Down syndrome, a form of mental retardation that occurs when a mistake in forming the eggs, or sometimes the sperm, leaves an additional chromosome in the fertilized egg. Individuals who have Down syndrome have an extra chromosome 21 (giving them three copies of chromosome 21 instead of two). They therefore have 47, instead of 46, chromosomes. Some disorders result from an incorrect arrangement of the chromosomal material (such as the loss of part of a chromosome). For all such disorders, there are many types of *microscope-based techniques* that can reveal the total chromosome number and permit the overall arrangement of the chromosomal material to be examined.

Biochemical Tests

For disorders brought on by flaws in individual genes, there are *biochemical techniques* that give information about the status of individual genes by measuring and scrutinizing the actual gene products, the proteins, that are present in body cells. Other biochemical procedures can look for specific changes in overall body chemistry that are known to come about because of defects in specific genes.

Biochemical techniques can measure the quantity of the protein that has been produced by the pair of genes responsible for that protein. The total amount of functional protein present can indicate whether any mutant genes are present. For example, the absence of one enzyme protein (officially hexosaminidase A, but called "hex-A" for short) causes the multiple and injurious features of Tay-Sachs disease, a lethal autosomal recessive genetic disorder. Babies with the disorder have inherited two defective copies of the gene for this protein and produce no functional enzyme. They die in early childhood due to problems arising from the absence of the enzyme. Carriers, those individuals with one normal and one defective gene, produce only half as much of the enzyme. This amount still provides more than enough functional protein so that carriers of the mutation have no adverse health effects. Biochemical tests that reveal a reduced level of the hex-A enzyme allow the carriers, who otherwise have no symptoms of any kind, to be identified and distinguished from noncarriers—those who possess two functional genes and produce high levels of the enzyme.

For some genetic disorders, the protein product is made, but it has somewhat altered properties because of a mutation in the DNA of the gene that produces it. The presence of such proteins with altered properties can often be picked up through the use of biochemical procedures. Examples of disorders that can be detected in this way are those involving the hemoglobin molecule, which transports oxygen through-out the body, and the collagen molecule, which provides structural sup-port throughout the body.

Biochemical tests have been employed for a very long time and are the first tests ordered when illnesses—genetic or otherwise—are being diagnosed. A wide array of biochemical procedures can be used to check if the overall cell chemistry has been thrown askew by a genetic or other malfunction. For example, hemochromatosis, a genetic condition in which excess amounts of iron accumulate in the blood and are stored in body organs, can first be detected through simple blood tests that measure blood iron levels.

DNA Tests

Laboratory techniques now make it possible to go beyond looking at whole chromosomes or measuring the protein products of specific genes. These are techniques that can examine the DNA itself. They are capable of locking onto places in or near the DNA of a specific gene and of examining certain features of that gene. These new capabilities in laboratory techniques have led to revolutionary changes in genetic testing. DNA tests are the key features of genetic medicine.

A *direct test* can recognize the tiny alterations or mutations that change the instructions contained in the DNA of a gene. These are the very changes that damage the gene's ability to function properly. Changes in the DNA sequence of the gene—even by one base pair—can be detected. If the mutation is one in which short sequences of bases are repeated over and over again, the presence and number of the repeats can be assessed. Thus direct DNA tests can disclose precise details of a gene's DNA base sequence.

The power of these direct DNA tests to reveal the status of genes is extraordinary. But there are limits. A direct DNA test can be done only when it is known what specific gene is involved in the genetic disorder. And, most often, not only must the gene be known, but the specific flaws within the DNA of that gene that cause it to malfunction must also be known. For instance, direct tests can be done to see if the single mutation responsible for sickle-cell anemia is present. The value of the direct test is diminished if the gene is a very long one and there are so many different possible mutations within it that it is not practical to test for each one. In such a case, the direct test can be designed to look for the most common mutations, but not rare or unusual ones. Direct tests of the gene associated with cystic fibrosis can pick up 90 percent of the mutations. This means that there will still be people who have mutations that the test cannot detect.

If there is, at present, no clue about what the gene itself is, what changes occur in its DNA sequence, or what its function is, there is another type of DNA test that can be used. This is the *linkage test*. What happens in a linkage test is this: When there is no way to detect the "target" gene directly, a known region of DNA located close to the target gene can be used as a "marker" for the target gene. By following the marker, predictions about the actual state of the nearby target gene can be made. The marker serves as an indicator in much the same way that a buoy floating on the surface of the water warns sailors of a hidden hazard located below the surface.

Linkage testing is more complicated than direct DNA testing for two reasons. First, it requires information about which markers are adjacent to the target genes on both chromosomes. The nature of the markers found on the chromosomes can differ from family to family. This means that several family members—especially those members who have the genetic disorder in question—need to be tested to figure out which marker is traveling along with the mutant gene and which with the normal gene. It is also necessary that the marker that travels along with the mutant gene be different from the marker that travels along with the normal gene. If the two markers are identical, then there is no way to distinguish the mutant from the normal gene. And, second, even when the genetic conditions are right for linkage analysis to be attempted, one has to be cautious when drawing conclusions from the results. What is really happening in linkage testing is the making of informed guesses (or predictions) based on a region of DNA at a short distance from the actual target gene. Regions of DNA can sometimes be exchanged between chromosomes. It can occasionally happen that the markers will have been switched. (The farther apart they are, the more opportunity there is for switching to occur.) The marker originally linked up with the mutant gene will now be attached to the normal gene, and vice versa. As a result, linkage testing cannot give an absolutely certain answer about whether a particular gene is present. What it can provide is the likelihood or *probability* that a particular form of a gene has been inherited along with its marker. A typical result of a genetic test for an autosomal dominant mutation might be stated in this way: there is a 95 percent chance that you have inherited the normal form of a gene and a 5 percent chance that you have inherited the mutant gene. Many genetic counselors prefer to present the results as "high risk" or "low risk" so that it is clear that some uncertainty remains.

Point 10: Genetic Tests Are Possible throughout the Life Cycle

Any type of genetic test requires a sample of tissue containing cells from the individual being tested. This usually involves taking a small amount of blood or dislodging some cells by rubbing the inside of the cheek with a cotton swab. To determine the genetic status of an individual who is no longer alive, it is sometimes possible to track down tissue samples held in pathology-lab archives and use a small portion for genetic testing.

Testing of the fetus, prior to birth, can be done using procedures that permit fetal cells to be accessed and collected. In one of these procedures, called *amniocentesis,* a sample of the amniotic fluid (the fluid surrounding the fetus) is collected. The fluid is drawn out using a needle inserted through the mother's abdominal wall and uterus and into the amniotic sac. For genetic testing purposes, this is generally done at about the sixteenth week of gestation. The amniotic fluid contains fetal cells that can be examined to reveal the status of the chromosomes, individual genes, and specific proteins. In another of these procedures, *chorionic villus sampling,* cells on the outside of the chorionic sac (the outermost covering surrounding the fetus) are collected from about the tenth to the twelfth week of gestation. Both means of gathering fetal cells carry with them a small risk of complications that can ultimately bring about the termination of the pregnancy.

Newer techniques can gain genetic information even earlier, during the embryonic stage (the name given to the first eight weeks of gestation).

Preimplantation genetic diagnosis involves the use of reproductive technologies to fertilize the egg in the laboratory. Following fertilization, one or two cells from the early embryo can be removed and examined for the status of particular genes. If the mutant genes are absent, the remaining embryo can, remarkably, be implanted in the uterus to continue through gestation. The possibility of a successful pregnancy is reduced with this technique, because of the many manipulations that are involved. Currently, preimplantation genetic diagnosis is only used in special circumstances.

Despite the ease of collecting genetic material, one should not be led to believe that genetic testing is easily done or that it is a standard or normal part of medical care. Genetic testing can raise troubling personal and family and societal issues. Decisions about whether or not to have a genetic test require extremely careful consideration.

Glossary

amniocentesis A procedure usually carried out at about the sixteenth week of pregnancy that obtains a sample of the fluid (amniotic fluid) surrounding the fetus. The fluid is collected by insertion of a needle through the mother's abdominal wall and into the sac immediately surrounding the fetus. Studies of the fluid and the fetal cells contained within it can provide information about the fetus's chromosomes, genes, and chemical makeup.

autosomal dominant A pattern of inheritance attributed to genes located on chromosomes other than the X and Y (sex) chromosomes. The trait or disorder will appear even when only one copy of the gene for that trait or disorder is present. Males and females are equally likely to be affected, and the trait can show up in successive generations of a family.

autosomal recessive A pattern of inheritance attributed to genes located on chromosomes other than the X and Y (sex) chromosomes. Both copies of the gene in a gene pair must be flawed for a disorder to appear. Males and females are equally likely to be affected. The disorder can appear suddenly with no prior history of it in the family.

autosome Any chromosome that is not part of the pair of sex chromosomes. Humans have twenty-two pairs of autosomes, numbered from 1 to 22.

base Any one of the four units—adenine (A), guanine (G), thymine (T), and cytosine (C)—found in a DNA molecule. The order (sequence) of the bases along one strand of the DNA molecule provides information for assembling proteins. The bases on one DNA strand pair up with the bases on the other DNA strand (A with T, G with C), providing stability to the DNA molecule.

carrier An individual who has a gene pair in which one of the genes is flawed. The presence of the flawed gene is masked by the dominant functional gene.

carrier test A genetic test performed to determine if a healthy individual has a flawed gene that has no effect on that individual but, if paired up with a similar flawed gene in his or her partner, could lead to a genetic disorder in their child.

cell The basic building block of all organisms. The human body is composed of trillions of cells, specialized into many cell types including muscle, nerve, blood, bone, and skin cells.

chorionic villus sampling A procedure, usually carried out between the tenth and twelfth weeks of pregnancy, to collect cells from placental tissue. Samples can be taken in several ways. Studies of these cells can yield information about fetal chromosomes and genes.

chromosome A long ribbonlike structure containing collections of genes. The standard number of chromosomes in humans is forty-six.

complex disorder A disorder that arises out of a combination of genetic and environmental factors. Cancer, heart disease, diabetes, and many other common health problems fall into this category. (See also *multifactorial disorder*.)

direct test A test that can detect specific mutations or alterations in a gene.

DNA The abbreviation for deoxyribonucleic acid, the threadlike molecule that is the genetic material. DNA has the form of a double-stranded helix. Each strand contains a long sequence of four types of chemical bases (denoted as A, C, G, and T). The sequence of bases makes up the genetic code containing the information for all of the proteins that an organism can produce. The helix is held together by strand-to-strand bonds, following the chemical rule that A connects to T, and G connects to C. DNA is located in the chromosomes within the organism's cells.

dominant mutation A mutation whose effect is revealed even when it is present in only one of the genes in the gene pair. (See also *autosomal dominant*.)

enzyme protein A type of protein whose function is to act as a catalyst and make chemical reactions possible in living organisms. In the absence of the enzyme, the chemical reaction for which the enzyme is responsible will not take place.

eugenics The term given to public policies that attempt to improve human populations by promoting the reproduction of individuals having what are regarded as "good" genes and preventing the repro duction of individuals having so-called bad genes. Such policies were promoted in many different countries, including the United States. Eugenic policies fell into disrepute after the Second World War because of their lack of scientific validity and the clear evidence of their painful human cost.

family health history A collection of health information about individuals in a family group, often displayed in pictorial form, to allow patterns of illness to be recognized and the possible role of genetic factors to be considered.

gamete A male or female reproductive cell. In the female, an ovum (or egg); in the male, a sperm.

gene A defined section of DNA along the chromosome that encodes information for the production of a particular protein necessary for the functioning of the organism.

gene pair The two genes, one derived from each parent, with information for producing a protein. One gene comes from the chromosome set contributed by the egg cell, the other gene from the chromosome set contributed by the sperm cell. All genes come in pairs with the exception of genes on the X chromosome in males. Males have only one X chromosome, therefore the genes on the X chromosome in males are present only in a single dose.

genetic counseling A multifaceted interaction between a genetic professional and a client in which information about individual and family genetic risks is provided along with related information about tests, treatments, and reproductive options.

genetic test Any type of laboratory procedure or investigation that reveals the status of a person's chromosomes or of that person's genes.

genome The total genetic material contained in a full set of chromosomes of an organism.

health history (See *family health history*.)

hemoglobin The molecule that transports oxygen throughout the body. It is made up of four chains, two of one type of protein and two of another. Changes in either of the proteins can lead to impaired function, such as occurs in sickle-cell anemia.

karyotype An organized picture showing all of the chromosomes in a cell.

late-onset disorder A disorder that is not apparent at birth but develops later in the course of an individual's life.

linkage test An indirect form of genetic testing in which a known region of DNA located near a gene for a disorder can be used as a "marker"—or indicator—for that gene. This type of testing is used when the target gene has not yet been identified or when a direct test is not practical because the specific mutation is not known.

locus The position that a gene occupies on a chromosome.

Mendel's laws of inheritance The basic rules underlying the passage of traits from one generation to the next put forth in the mid-nineteenth century by an Austrian monk, Gregor Mendel, experimenting with pea plants. Mendel explained his data by proposing the existence of pairs of "factors" (later renamed "genes") that yield particular traits, the dominance of some factors over others, the separation of such factors during gamete formation, and the independent assortment of the factors associated with different traits. These ideas, now known as Mendel's laws, have been the foundation of modern genetics.

multifactorial disorder A disorder that is brought on by the joint action of multiple factors. The contributing factors include several different genes as well as various types of agents from the environment. (See also *complex disorder*.)

mutation Any permanent change or alteration in the genetic material, for example, in the DNA base sequence of a gene.

newborn screening Testing done shortly after birth to identify those babies who are destined to develop a genetic disorder in order to begin treatments, such as changes in diet, that will prevent or reduce the harmful consequences of that disorder.

noninformative result A situation arising in genetic testing in which, following the testing, no firm conclusions can be drawn.

nucleus The place within the cell where the chromosomes are contained. It is separated from the rest of the cell by a porous membrane.

pharmacogenomics The branch of genetics that seeks both to understand the genetic differences underlying different responses to medications and to develop drugs tailored to individual genetic differences.

predictive tests Genetic tests that are conducted in advance of any symptoms of a disorder. This term applies both to presymptomatic tests (in which the disorder will occur if the mutant gene is found) and susceptibility tests (in which one's risk for a disorder increases if the mutant gene is found).

preimplantation genetic diagnosis (PGD) A procedure in which genetic testing is performed on one or two cells removed from the early embryo. Only embryos found to be free of disease-causing genes would then be placed in a woman's uterus to achieve a pregnancy.

prenatal test A genetic test performed during pregnancy to obtain information about the chromosomes or genes of a fetus.

presymptomatic test A genetic test performed to determine if a gene or genes are present that will bring on a health problem later in an individual's life.

private mutation A mutation unique to a particular family.

probability The odds or chance that an event will happen. This is often expressed as a percentage. For example, a probability of 50% represents an event that is equally likely to happen as not to happen, an event that will happen half the time. A probability of 100% represents an event that is certain to happen. A probability of 0% represents an event that definitely will not happen.

prophylactic surgery The removal of healthy body organs—such as the thyroid gland, breasts, or ovaries—thereby reducing the possibility that any disease process affecting those organs can occur. This is also known as "risk-reduction" surgery.

protein A molecule composed of amino acids connected together in a linear fashion. The order (sequence) of the amino acids in a protein is determined by the order of bases found within the DNA of a gene.

recessive mutation A mutation whose effect is revealed only when it occurs in both genes of a gene pair. (See also *autosomal recessive*.)

regulatory proteins Proteins that help control the activities of genes or that integrate the different chemical processes that occur in an organism.

repeats or repeated sequences A series of two or more DNA bases that occurs over and over in tandem at one place on a chromosome. Some disorders (such as Huntington disease, fragile-X syndrome, and myotonic dystrophy) result when a three-base sequence (such as CAG in Huntington disease) recurs many times within a gene. In some cases, there can be an expansion in number of repeats in successive generations.

sequence The linear order of the bases in the DNA molecule or of amino acids in a protein molecule. The process of determining the actual order of bases in a gene is known as "sequencing."

sex chromosomes The X and Y chromosomes. Females have two X chromosomes; males have one X and one Y. (See also *X-linked dominant* and *X-linked recessive*.)

single-gene disorder A disorder that comes about when there is a mutation in a specific gene, and one (for a dominant disorder) or both (for a recessive disorder) of the genes in the gene pair cannot function properly.

somatic mutation A mutation that occurs in any of the body cells of an individual over the course of that person's life. Since the mutation is not in the eggs or the sperm cells, it cannot be passed on to children.

structural protein A type of protein whose function is to provide shape and support to the various parts of the organism.

susceptibility gene A gene that, when mutated, increases the changes that an individual will develop a disorder later on in his or her life. However, the disorder may not develop even if the damaged gene is present, and it may occur even in the absence of the mutation. Examples of such genes are the BRCA1 and BRCA2 genes which, when mutated, raise the risk of breast and/or ovarian cancer. (See *complex disorder*.)

susceptibility test A test for a gene mutation whose presence can increase the chances of developing a health problem later in life.

true negative An individual who can be shown, through genetic testing, not to have inherited a known mutation associated with a particular disorder.

X-linked dominant A pattern of inheritance attributed to genes located on the X chromosome. A disorder will appear when one copy of the gene for that disorder is present. Males can pass X-linked dominant genes to all of their daughters but none of their sons. Females pass X-linked dominant genes, on average, to half of their daughters and half of their sons.

X-linked recessive A pattern of inheritance attributed to genes located on the X chromosome. In males, all of whom have a single X chromosome, any recessive gene will be expressed. Thus, if a recessive gene for a disorder is present, the disorder will develop. In females, all of whom have two X chromosomes, a recessive gene for a disorder on one X chromosome can be masked by a functional gene on the other X chromosome. Such females, while healthy themselves, pass X-linked recessive genes, on average, to half of their sons (who then develop the disorder) and to half of their daughters (who then become carriers like their mother).

Resources

The information listed in this section can change over time. A link to a continuously updated list of these resources can be found on the Internet at http://www.sts.vt.edu/totestornot.

How to Develop a Family Health History

Any of the following books and Web sites should provide a good starting point for putting together one's own family health history.

Books

Gormley, Myra Vanderpool. 1998. *Family Diseases: Are You at Risk?* Baltimore: Genealogical Publishing Co.

Jerger, Jeanette. 1999. *A Medical Miscellany for Genealogists*. Bowie, MD: Heritage Books, Inc. This reference book can help connect the common names for various diseases with their medical equivalents.

Krause, Carol. 1995. *How Healthy Is Your Family Tree: A Complete Guide to Tracing Your Family's Medical and Behavioral History*. New York: Simon & Schuster.

Nelson-Anderson, Danette, and Cynthia Waters. 1995. *Genetic Connections: A Guide to Documenting Your Individual and Family Health History*. Washington, MO: Sonters Publishing. This book can be ordered through the following Web site: http://pages.prodigy. net/sydrs/.

Web Sites

American Medical Association
http://www.ama-assn.org/ama/pub/category/2380.html

This site includes several questionnaires that can guide information collection in a way that makes it particularly helpful to your physician or genetic counselor. A pamphlet, *Family Medical History in Disease Prevention*, is also available at this Web site. Although intended for physicians, it has links to resources on how to collect family health information and how to generate a simple pedigree that make it useful for consumers as well.

Genetic Alliance
http://www.geneticalliance.org. Click on the "Family Health History" link at the bottom to reach *Does It Run in the Family? A Guide to Family Health History*. This document is a collaborative effort of the American Folklife Center, the American Society of Human Genetics, the Genetic Alliance, and the Institute for Cultural Partnerships.

Genetics Education and Outreach Network
http://www.genednet.org/pages/consumer_family.shtml

Mayo Clinic
http://www.mayoclinic.com/health/medical-history/HQ01707/
UPDATEAPP=0

National Genealogical Society, The Family Health and Hereditary Committee
http://www.ngsgenealogy.org/comfamhealth.cfm

National Society of Genetic Counselors
http://www.nsgc.org/consumer/familytree/index.cfm

Oprah.com
http://www.oprah.com/omagazine/200504/omag_200504_tree.jhtml

U.S. Department of Health and Human Services
http://www.hhs.gov/familyhistory. These materials were developed as part of the Surgeon General's Family History Initiative. Family health information collected at this Web site can be printed out as a diagram or in chart form so that it can be shared with other family members and with family physicians.

http://www.hhs.gov/familyhistory/download.html. Software, in English and Spanish, is available at this site and can be downloaded to personal computers.

University of Utah, Utah Department of Health, Health Family Tree http://health.utah.gov/genomics/familyhistory/toolkit.html. Free printed copies of this toolkit can be obtained by calling the Health Resource Line at 1–888–222–2542.

Where to Learn More about Genetics

A genetics tutorial can be found in the appendix to this book.

The books and Web sites listed below are useful for gaining greater insight into human genetics and its medical applications.

Books

Hartl, Daniel L., and Elizabeth W. Jones. 2006. *Essential Genetics: A Genomics Perspective*. 4th ed. Sudbury, MA: Jones and Bartlett.

Lewis, Ricki. 2007. *Human Genetics, Concepts and Applications*. 7th ed. New York: McGraw-Hill.

Maroni, Gustavo. 2001. *Molecular and Genetic Analysis of Human Traits*. Malden, MA: Blackwell Science.

Read, Andrew, and Dian Donnai. 2007. *New Clinical Genetics*. Bloxham, Oxfordshire, UK: Scion.

Witherly, Jeffre, Galen P. Perry, and Darryl L. Leja. 2001. *An A to Z of DNA Science: What Scientists Mean When They Talk about Genes and Genomes*. Cold Spring Harbor, NY: Cold Spring Harbor Laboratory Press.

The following books may be of particular interest to health professionals:

Bennett, Robin L. 1999. *The Practical Guide to the Genetic Family History*. New York: Oxford University Press.

Harper, Peter S. 2004. *Practical Genetic Counseling*. 6th ed. Hodder Arnold.

King, Richard A., Jerome I. Rotter, and Arno G. Motulsky. 2002. *The Genetic Basis of Common Diseases*. 2nd ed. New York: Oxford University Press.

Nussbaum, Robert, Roderick R. McInnes, and Huntington F. Willard. 2007. *Thompson & Thompson Genetics in Medicine.* 7th ed. St. Louis: Elsevier.

Offit, K., J. Garber, M. Grady, M. H. Greene, S. Gruber, B. Peshkin, M. Rodriguez-Bigas, J. Trimbath, and J. Weitzel. 2004. *ASCO Curriculum: Cancer Genetics and Cancer Predisposition Testing.* 2nd ed. Alexandria, VA: ASCO.

Pasternak, Jack J. 2005. *An Introduction to Human Molecular Genetics: Mechanisms of Inherited Diseases.* 2nd ed. Hoboken, NJ: Wiley Interscience.

Skirton, Heather. 2005. *Applied Genetics in Healthcare: A Handbook for Specialist Practitioners.* New York and Oxford: Taylor and Francis.

Web Sites

About.com
http://biology.about.com/od/basicgenetics/a/aa071705a.htm

GlaxoSmithKline. *Introduction to Genetics*
http://genetics.gsk.com/overview.htm

Howard Hughes Medical Institute. *Blazing a Genetic Trail*
http://www.hhmi.org/genetictrail

NIH: National Cancer Institute, Understanding Cancer Series
http://www.cancer.gov/cancertopics/understandingcancer/genetesting

U.S. Department of Energy Human Genome Program. *Genomics and Its Impact on Medicine and Society: The Human Genome Project and Beyond* (2003).
http://www.ornl.gov/sci/techresources/Human_Genome/publicat/primer/index.shtml

U.S. Department of Health and Human Services. *Understanding Genetic Testing.*
http://www.accessexcellence.org/AE/AEPC/NIH/index.html

U.S. National Library of Medicine Handbook, *Help Me Understand Genetics.*
http://ghr.nlm.nih.gov/handbook

Ways to Obtain Basic Information about Health Problems

Contact a Family, a U.K. charity for families with children who are disabled
http://www.cafamily.org.uk/home.html. The Contact a Family directory contains information on common and rare disorders affecting children and adults.

GeneTests, University of Washington, Seattle
http://www.geneclinics.org/profiles

National Organization for Rare Disorders (NORD)
http://www.rarediseases.org/search/rdblist.html. Despite its name, the NORD Web site contains information about many common disorders as well as rare disorders.

U.S. Department of Health and Human Services
http://www.healthfinder.gov

U.S. National Institutes of Health
http://health.nih.gov

Genetics and Rare Diseases Information Center, NIH Office of Rare Diseases
http://rarediseases.info.nih.gov/asp/diseases/diseases.asp

U.S. National Library of Medicine
http://www.nlm.nih.gov/medlineplus/healthtopics.html
http://ghr.nlm.nih.gov/ghr/page/BrowseConditions. This site contains information on genetic conditions.

The following organizations provide information about the specific disorders that served as the main examples in this book.

Alzheimers Association
http://alz.org/alzheimers_disease_what_is_alzheimers.asp

Alzheimer's Disease Education and Referral Center (ADEAR)
http://www.nia.nih.gov/Alzheimers

American Academy of Family Physicians: Hereditary Hemochromatosis
http://familydoctor.org/online/famdocen/home/common/blood/758.
html

American Cancer Society
National Headquarters
1599 Clifton Road, N.E.
Atlanta, Georgia 30329
(800) ACS-2345 (toll free)
http://www.cancer.org

Cancerbackup, Cancer Information Charity, U.K.
Free phone helpline: 0808 800 1234
http://www.cancerbackup.org.uk/Home

Cancer Information Service
(800) 4-CANCER (toll free). This is a national toll-free telephone
inquiry system that, according to its charter, "provides information
about cancer and cancer-related resources to the general public,
patients and their families, as well as health professionals."

U.S. National Institutes of Health Cancer Net
http://www.cancer.gov. This site also includes links to clinical
trials.

Ways to Find Genetic Professionals in Your Area

To locate genetics professionals, contact any of the following organizations. Where noted, there are also links to international organizations.

Genetic Interest Group, U.K.
http://www.gig.org.uk/services.htm. This site contains a directory of
genetic centers and services throughout the U.K.

GeneTests, University of Washington, Seattle
http://www.geneclinics.org. Click on "Clinic Directory" for links to
U.S.-based and international clinics.

National Society of Genetic Counselors
http://www.nsgc.org. Click on the "Find a Counselor" link.

U.S. National Institutes of Health, Cancer Genetics Services Directory
http://www.cancer.gov/search/genetics_services

Ways to Find Support Groups

Support groups for specific conditions can be identified by contacting
the following umbrella organizations.

Genetic Alliance
4301 Connecticut Ave. NW, Suite 404
Washington, DC 20008–2369
Main office: (202) 966–5557
(202) 966–8553 (fax)
E-mail: info@geneticalliance.org
http://www.geneticalliance.org. Click on "Organization Search"

Making Contact.Org, A Service of Contact a Family, UK
http://www.makingcontact.org. This site is geared toward helping
families with disabled children reach out to one another. Several language options are available.

MUMS: National Parent-to-Parent Network
Julie J. Gordon
150 Custer Court
Green Bay, WI 54301–1243
(877) 336–5333 (for parents only)
(920) 336–5333
(920) 339–0995 (fax)
E-mail: mums@netnet.net
http://www.netnet.net/mums/database.htm

National Organization for Rare Disorders (NORD)
http://www.rarediseases.org/search/orglist.html

University of Kansas Medical Center
http://www.kumc.edu/gec/support/index.html. This Web site can
direct consumers to national and international organizations.

Links to some support groups for the disorders that served as the examples in this book.

Alzheimer's Association
225 N. Michigan Ave., Fl. 17
Chicago, IL 60601–7633
(312) 335–8700
(312) 335–5886 (TDD)
(866) 699–1246 (fax)
24/7 helpline for information, referral, and support: (800) 272–3900 (toll free); (866) 403–3073 (TDD)
E-mail: info@alz.org
http://www.alz.org. Click on "In My Community" to search for organizations in your area.

American Hemochromatosis Society
4044 W. Lake Mary Blvd., Unit #104, PMB 416
Lake Mary, FL 32746
(407) 829–4488
(407) 333–1284 (fax)
24-hour information hotline: (888) 655–IRON (4766) (toll free)
http://americanhs.org

Canadian Hemochromatosis Society
7000 Minoru Blvd., Suite 272
Richmond, BC, Canada V6Y 3Z5
(877) BAD–IRON, or (877) 223–4766 (toll free)
(604) 279–7135
(604) 279–7138 (fax)
E-mail: office@toomuchiron.ca
http://www.toomuchiron.ca

Colon Cancer Alliance
1200 G Street, NW, Suite 800
Washington, DC 20005
(866) 304–9075 (fax)

(877) 422–2030 (helpline)
http://www.ccalliance.org

FORCE: Facing Our Risk of Cancer Empowered (for individuals concerned about hereditary breast and/or ovarian cancer)
16057 Tampa Palms Blvd. W, PMB #373
Tampa, FL 33647
(954) 255–8732
(954) 827–2200 (fax)
(866) 288–RISK (toll-free voice mail)
E-mail: info@facingourrisk.org
(866) 824–RISK (7475) (toll-free helpline)
http://www.facingourrisk.org

Some Additional Resources That May Be of Interest

Equal Employment Opportunities Commission
1801 L Street, NW
Washington, DC 20507
(202) 419–0713
(800) 800–3302 (TDD)
This is the federal agency that oversees the employment provisions of
the Americans with Disabilities Act. You may be referred on to another
federal agency or to a state agency based on the nature of your request.

National Conference of State Legislatures
http://www.ncsl.org/programs/health/genetics/charts.htm. This site
contains current information about the laws dealing with genetics that
are in force in each state.

PubMed
http://www.nlm.nih.gov/pubs/factsheets/pubmed.html. This site, a
collaborative effort of the U.S. National Library of Medicine and the
National Institutes of Health, allows free public access to a vast scientific and medical literature.

Tutorials are available to allow this site to be used most effectively.
These tutorials can be found at http://www.nlm.nih.gov/bsd/
disted/pubmed.html#qt.

Index

Page numbers in boldface refer to glossary entries.

About the Author

Doris Teichler Zallen is a professor in the Department of Science and Technology in Society at Virginia Tech. Educated as a biologist (B.S., Brooklyn College; Ph.D., Harvard), her early work focused on cell biology and genetics. Her research now centers on the ethical, social, and policy issues raised by advances in genetic science, especially genetic testing. She is the founder of the award-winning *Choices and Challenges* public humanities educational project and is a past member of the NIH Recombinant DNA Advisory Committee (the "RAC"), where she helped provide oversight of ground-breaking human gene-therapy experiments. While on the RAC, she worked to establish better protections for the human subjects of that research. In 2007, she received an Outstanding Faculty Award from the Commonwealth of Virginia.